EDGAR CAYCE'S
DIET
AND
RECIPE GUIDE

EDGAR CAYCE'S
DIET
AND
RECIPE GUIDE

by the Editors of A.R.E. Press

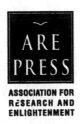

ARE PRESS

ASSOCIATION FOR
RESEARCH AND
ENLIGHTENMENT

A.R.E. Press • Virginia Beach • Virginia

A.R.E. Press
215 67th Street
Virginia Beach, VA 23451-2061

Library of Congress Cataloging-in-Publication Data
Edgar Cayce's diet and recipe guide / by the editors of A.R.E. Press
    p. cm.
This book is a compilation of two booklets originally published by
A.R.E. Press during the 1950s and '60s, which have been republished
for the new millennium. The first, called The normal diet, was origi-
nally published in 1957 and was selected and arranged by Margaret
Gammon; the second booklet, A diet recipe guide based on the Edgar
Cayce readings by Ann Read and Carol Ilstrup, was first published in
1967.
    Includes index.
    ISBN 0-87604-414-3
    1. Nutrition. I. Cayce, Edgar, 1877-1945. II. Read, Anne. Edgar
Cayce on diet and health. III. Association for Research and Enlightenment. IV. Diet recipe guide based on the Edgar Cayce
readings.
RA784.E315 1999
613.2—dc21   98-21748

Cover design by Lightbourne

Contents

INTRODUCTION

Many individuals become aware of the physical benefits others have gained through the readings of Edgar Cayce and
lament the fact that a personal reading from Mr. Cayce is no
longer possible. The question then arises, "Can I benefit from
the information given for others in the past?" or "Can information given through Edgar Cayce for an individual with a specific
condition be used by another whose physical condition is different?"

While it is true that much of the content of the physical readings applies only to specific individuals, there are a number of
readings that may apply to all. This is especially true of the recommendations on diet, since many of these readings contain
statements such as "This would be well for all" or "as with most
physical bodies." Much of the information is frequently repeated, indicating universal relevance. The material in this book
is based upon that information which seems beneficial to any-
one seeking a basic, healthy diet.

This book is a compilation of two booklets first published by
A.R.E. Press during the 1950s and '60s. The first booklet, *The Normal Diet*, was originally published in 1957 and was selected and
arranged by Margaret Gammon, who at the time had worked in
the area of food and nutrition for over fifteen years. It is filled
with quotes from the readings and guidelines for following
Cayce's normal diet. The second booklet, *A Diet Recipe Guide
Based on the Edgar Cayce Readings* by Ann Read and Carol
Ilstrup, was first published in 1967. It is primarily a collection of
recipes designed to complement the normal diet.

The original compilation of this material from the Cayce readings has a high degree of conformance with the prevailing dietetic opinion of its day. The recipes are in keeping with these concepts.

Many changes, however, in what science knows about diet and nutrition have occurred since the original booklets were written. As a result of new dietary information, in 1992 the U.S. Department of Agriculture (USDA) adopted the Food Guide Pyramid, which was designed to replace the outdated Basic 7 food groups as a guide for normal daily diet. The Food Guide Pyramid appears in this book.

Much has changed in the availability and quality of ingredients since the original recipes were published in the late 1950s and '60s. There has also been an increased awareness regarding saturated fat, cholesterol, and other dietary red flags. Readers concerned about high cholesterol, for example, may want to exercise prudence with recipes that use large quantities of eggs or other ingredients high in cholesterol. Nevertheless, the recipes have been left intact but contain nutritional updates and, where appropriate, new product options for substituting ingredients.

Almost everyone who consulted Edgar Cayce for physical readings, given between 1901 and his death in 1945, was given dietary suggestions. This focus on diet, even for those who did not request dietary information, shows the interrelatedness of the body, mind, and soul. The original booklets concerned the normal diet for healthy people. As such, all dietary suggestions for people with physical ailments—even constipation and obesity, common as they are—were eliminated. They remain absent from this volume as well. Information on Cayce's dietary recommendations for those who are ill and his readings on other health-related topics are available from the Association for Research and Enlightenment, Inc., 215 67th Street, Virginia Beach, VA 23451-2061.

The greatest strength of this book is that it shares the dietary information from the Edgar Cayce readings that has proved beneficial over the years in the lives of thousands of people worldwide.

—The Editors of A.R.E. Press

1

The Edgar Cayce Philosophy and the Normal Diet

*I*n the Edgar Cayce readings, the spiritual and mental life are not separated from the physical. All three are one, the readings gave. The importance of treating the body considerately, even reverently, since it is the temple of the spirit, is stressed over and over in the readings.

> The body of each entity is the temple of the living God . . . To live, to be—and that activity—unto the glory of the Creative Forces is the purpose of the entrance of each entity into material consciousness.   2981-1

> Study, then, those charts pertaining to keeping well balanced in the chemical forces; not as to become a human pillbox but rather knowing the law and keeping same.   2981-2

> There is as much of God in the physical as there is in the spiritual or mental, for it should be one!   69-5

> . . . each soul is as the temple of the living God . . . Thus be mindful more, not of the body for body's sake, but of the body that the temple of the living God may be the better channel for

the manifesting of the spiritual truths . . .   2938-1

Urges arise, then, not only from what one eats but from what one thinks; and from what one does about what one thinks and eats! as well as what one digests mentally and spiritually!   2533-6

Mind is ever the builder. That which the body-mind feeds upon, that it gradually becomes; provided that fed to the mind is assimilated by the mind body. Just as in the physical—without the activity of digestion, of assimilation. These are quite different in a physical body; that is: Digestion does not necessarily mean that what is digested is assimilated. Neither in the mental body does it mean that what is read, heard or spoken to the body, is assimilated by the mental body.   3102-1

There only needs be that the body keep that diet . . . that the physical needs through its inmost desires, and not override those conditions by the will of the individual. For the inmost conditions of desire in the individual would and do lead the physical of this body correctly. Only when these are overridden by the self-aggrandizement, or self motives of the carnal excess, or success of the physical, does the body become enamoured with these conditions that hinder . . . Keep in those lines that lead to the understanding of self, and so present the physical that it may be holy and acceptable unto Him; remembering that the physical is the earthly temple of the God to whom one should give of one's best, and it is only a reasonable service that this be presented holy and acceptable unto Him.   257-6

What effect have the emotions upon digestion and assimilation? A direct effect, the readings declare:

. . . being mindful of the diets that they are kept proper. Take *time* to eat and to eat the right thing, giving time for digestive forces [to act] before becoming so mentally and bodily active as to upset digestion.   243-23

True, the body should eat—and should eat slowly; yet when worried, overtaxed, or when the body may not make a *business* of the eating, but eating to pass away the time, or just to fill up time, not good—for, it *will not* digest, as the body sees. 900-393

Especially to this body there should not be food taken when the body is overwrought in any manner, whether of highstrung conditions or that of wrath, or of depressions of any nature. Food should not be taken in the system at such times; preferably take water, or buttermilk—*never* sweet milk under such conditions.
                                                                243-7

To overload the stomach when the body is worried, or under any general strain, is a great *detriment* to the better physical functioning. To make for the taking of foods whether there is felt the need or desire of same is equally as bad for the body. 277-1

... *never*, under strain, when very tired, very excited, very mad, should the body take foods in the system ... And never take any food that the body finds is not agreeing with same ...   137-30

What is a good everyday diet that will promote good health and keep the individual as a body, mind, and spirit unit functioning on a high level? We are not born with this knowledge; we must learn it. The Edgar Cayce readings contribute a great deal to our understanding.

For the purpose of comparison, consider the food groups listed in the USDA Food Guide Pyramid (see page 5). We are encouraged to choose in suggested quantities from these groups each day. By doing this, we obtain food elements that (1) yield energy, (2) supply materials for growth, and (3) keep the body in good running order. Here is the list of categories in the Food Guide Pyramid:

1. Bread, Cereal, Rice and Pasta Group—6 to 11 servings daily
2. Vegetable Group—3 to 5 servings daily
3. Fruit Group—2 to 4 servings daily
4. Milk, Yogurt, and Cheese Group—2 to 3 servings daily
5. Meat, Poultry, Fish, Dry Beans, Eggs, and Nuts Group—2 to 3 servings daily
6. Fats, Oils, and Sweets—use sparingly

While the Edgar Cayce readings do not classify foods into such a food pyramid or even the old Basic 7 scheme, they do agree with the ideal of variety and balance in the daily food elements. The readings emphasize certain ideas about to daily food selections, from which we can list these seven points:

1. Eat more fruits and vegetables
2. Watch the acid-alkaline balance in the body
3. Avoid certain food combinations
4. Keep a balance between foods grown above and below ground
5. Eat lightly of heavy meats; use fish, fowl, and lamb, plus eggs and milk
6. Use whole grain cereals and grains
7. Avoid fried foods; use fat sparingly

For a more in-depth view of Cayce's basic dietary recommendations, refer to the Basic Diet chart on page 7.

Before citing extracts from the readings to illustrate the above points and compare them with the Food Guide Pyramid, it is important to note that each reading covered a wide scope. There is a "spill over" of subject matter in each reading that is not only interesting to correlate but more helpful than when each point is considered separately.

Acid-Alkaline Balance

Balance is be a key word in the Cayce readings. We should strive to keep a balance of activities, attitudes, and the chemical composition of our bodies. One of the most important of these chemical balances is that of acidity and alkalinity.

The readings recognize the fact that a normal diet may vary among individuals, as some are more active than others. Most vegetables are alkaline-reacting; so are most fruits except prunes and cranberries. The readings give the ideal balance, as follows:

(Q) What should the diet be?
(A) Those things that will not create too much of an acid, or too much of an alkaline condition throughout the system. Rather

The Food Guide Pyramid

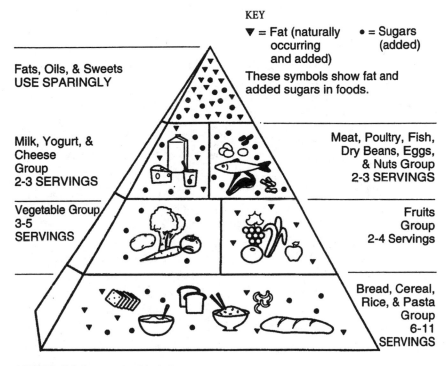

KEY

▼ = Fat (naturally occurring and added)   ● = Sugars (added)

These symbols show fat and added sugars in foods.

Fats, Oils, & Sweets
USE SPARINGLY

Milk, Yogurt, &
Cheese
Group
2-3 SERVINGS

Meat, Poultry, Fish,
Dry Beans, Eggs,
& Nuts Group
2-3 SERVINGS

Vegetable Group
3-5
SERVINGS

Fruits
Group
2-4 Servings

Bread, Cereal,
Rice, & Pasta
Group
6-11
SERVINGS

SOURCE: U.S. Department of Agriculture

be the alkaline than acid . . .   140-12

. . . in all bodies, the less activities there are in physical exercise or manual activity, the greater should be the alkaline-reacting foods taken. *Energies* or activities may burn acids, but those
who lead the sedentary life or the non-active life can't go on
sweets or too much starches—but these should be well-balanced.   798-1

(Q) What foods are acid-forming for this body?
(A) All of those that are combining fats with sugars. Starches
naturally are inclined for acid reaction. But a normal diet is about
twenty percent acid to eighty percent alkaline-producing.   1523-3

. . . have rather a percentage of eighty percent alkaline-producing to twenty percent acid-producing foods.
    Then, it is well that the body not become as one that couldn't
do this, that or the other; or as a slave to an idea of a set diet.
    Do not take citrus fruit juices *and* cereals at the same meal.
Do not take milk or cream in coffee or in tea. Do not eat fried
foods of any kind. Do not combine white bread, potatoes, spaghetti—or any two foods of such natures in the same meal.
                                                       1568-2

As indicated, keep a tendency for alkalinity in the diet. This
does not necessitate that there should *never* be any of the acid-
forming foods included in the diet; for an overalkalinity is much
more harmful than a little tendency occasionally for acidity. But
remember there are those tendencies in the system for cold and
congestion . . . and cold *cannot—does not—*exist in alkalines.
                                                       808-3

The diet should be more body-building; that is, less acid foods
and more of the alkaline-reacting . . . Milk and all its products
should be a portion of the body's diet now; also those food values carrying an easy assimilation of iron, silicon, and those elements or chemicals—as all forms of berries, most all forms of
vegetables that grow under the ground, most of the vegetables
of a leafy nature. Fruits and vegetables, nuts and the like, should

> "... what we think and what we eat—combined together— make *what we are; physically and mentally*."
>
> 288-38

Basic Diet

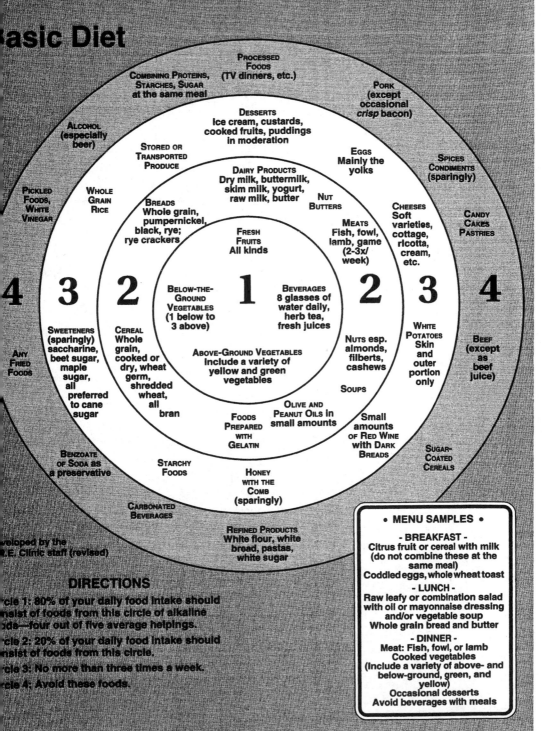

Circle 1 (center):
FRESH FRUITS All kinds

BELOW-THE-GROUND VEGETABLES (1 below to 3 above)

BEVERAGES 8 glasses of water daily, herb tea, fresh juices

1

ABOVE-GROUND VEGETABLES Include a variety of yellow and green vegetables

FOODS PREPARED WITH GELATIN

OLIVE AND PEANUT OILS in small amounts

HONEY WITH THE COMB (sparingly)

Circle 2:
DAIRY PRODUCTS Dry milk, buttermilk, skim milk, yogurt, raw milk, butter

NUT BUTTERS

BREADS Whole grain, pumpernickel, black, rye; rye crackers

MEATS Fish, fowl, lamb, game (2-3x/week)

CEREAL Whole grain, cooked or dry, wheat germ, shredded wheat, all bran

NUTS esp. almonds, filberts, cashews

SOUPS

Small amounts OF RED WINE with DARK BREADS

STARCHY FOODS

Circle 3:
STORED OR TRANSPORTED PRODUCE

DESSERTS Ice cream, custards, cooked fruits, puddings in moderation

EGGS Mainly the yolks

WHOLE GRAIN RICE

CHEESES Soft varieties, cottage, ricotta, cream, etc.

SWEETENERS (sparingly) saccharine, beet sugar, maple sugar, all preferred to cane sugar

WHITE POTATOES Skin and outer portion only

SUGAR-COATED CEREALS

CARBONATED BEVERAGES

Circle 4:
COMBINING PROTEINS, STARCHES, SUGAR at the same meal

PROCESSED FOODS (TV dinners, etc.)

PORK (except occasional *crisp* bacon)

ALCOHOL (especially beer)

SPICES CONDIMENTS (sparingly)

PICKLED FOODS, WHITE VINEGAR

CANDY CAKES PASTRIES

ANY FRIED FOODS

BEEF (except as beef juice)

BENZOATE OF SODA as a preservative

REFINED PRODUCTS White flour, white bread, pastas, white sugar

4   3   2   1   2   3   4

Developed by the A.R.E. Clinic staff (revised)

DIRECTIONS

Circle 1: 80% of your daily food intake should consist of foods from this circle of alkaline foods—four out of five average helpings.

Circle 2: 20% of your daily food intake should consist of foods from this circle.

Circle 3: No more than three times a week.

Circle 4: Avoid these foods.

• MENU SAMPLES •

- BREAKFAST -
Citrus fruit or cereal with milk (do not combine these at the same meal)
Coddled eggs, whole wheat toast

- LUNCH -
Raw leafy or combination salad with oil or mayonnaise dressing and/or vegetable soup
Whole grain bread and butter

- DINNER -
Meat: Fish, fowl, or lamb
Cooked vegetables
(Include a variety of above- and below-ground, green, and yellow)
Occasional desserts
Avoid beverages with meals

form a greater part of the regular diet in the present . . .

Keep closer to the alkaline diets; using fruits, berries, vegetables particularly that carry iron, silicon, phosphorus and the like . . .   480-19

. . . when there is the tendency towards an alkaline system there is less effect of cold and congestion.   270-33

Though "an overalkalinity is much more harmful than a little tendency occasionally for acidity" (808-3), apparently it is much rarer, the emphasis throughout being on more of alkaline-reacting foods.

In response to a question concerning common contagious diseases, this answer was given:

. . . if an alkalinity is maintained in the system—especially with lettuce, carrots and celery, these in the blood supply will maintain such a condition as to immunize a person.   480-19

Colds are often the result, according to the readings, of an unbalancing of the alkalinity of the system:

. . . cold *cannot—does not*—exist in alkalines.   808-3

Cayce recommended a balance of "about twenty percent acid to eighty percent alkaline-producing" (1523-3)—sufficiently alkaline yet not too much so.

Overacidity may be produced by overeating sweets, especially before sufficient food has been eaten at meals: "The acidity was produced by taking too much sugar in the system in candies, and in those properties as were taken before the stomach was filled with foods; and then overloading the system at such times . . . " (294-86) Also named as possible causes of overacidity were combining sweets and starches (340-32) and taking several starches at the same meal (416-18).

An abundance of vegetables and fruits, especially citrus fruits, helps to maintain the alkalinity of the system. Lemons, especially, are a good alkalizer, and the readings consistently recommend adding a little lemon or lime juice to orange juice.

(See 2072-3.) Vegetables should be in the proportions of three that grow above the ground to one that grows below the ground, and one leafy vegetable to every one of the pod vegetables.

Bernard Jensen, D.C., N.D., author, lecturer, and director of Hidden Valley Health Ranch at Escondido, California, during the 1960s, was in complete agreement with the Cayce readings as to both the importance of maintaining this balance and the proportions of different types of foods necessary to create the eighty percent alkaline and twenty percent acid balance. The correct proportions would be four vegetables and two fruits to one protein and one starch, he says, though he did not recommend keeping these exact proportions each day but rather approximating them over a period of time.

Dr. Jensen related two experiments that involved the effect of low acidity in the body. In one, turpentine was injected into the leg of a rabbit while it was alkalinized, with very slight damage resulting to the leg. The same amount of turpentine injected into the leg when the rabbit was acidized, however, resulted in inflammation, tissue sloughing, and death. In the other experiment it was discovered that among a number of scarlet fever patients, two-thirds of those with high acidity developed nephritis, while this complication occurred in only three percent of the cases in which the acidity was low.

When citrus fruits (which are strongly alkaline producing) cause distress, Dr. Jensen stated, it may be due to their tendency to stir up acids already accumulated in the body, giving the mistaken impression that they are having a bad effect.

In general, starchy foods, fatty foods, sugar (either white or raw), and proteins are acid forming, while fruits and vegetables are alkaline forming (with a few exceptions). Also, as Dr. Jensen pointed out, vegetables that are alkaline forming when fresh may become acid forming within a few days after being picked. Incorrect combinations of foods, according to the readings, become a factor in producing an overacid condition.

Acid-Forming Foods

Meats: beef, pork, lamb, veal
Poultry: chicken, turkey, duck, goose, guinea hen, game

Visceral meats: heart, brains, kidney, liver, sweetbreads, thymus
Egg whites (yolks are not acid forming)
Animal fats and vegetable oils
White sugar and syrups made from white sugar
Nuts: peanuts, English walnuts, pecans, filberts, coconut
Certain fruits, including large prunes, plums, and cranberries
Certain vegetables, including legumes (dried peas, dried beans, and lentils) and rhubarb
All cereal grains and other such products, like bread, breakfast foods, rolled oats, corn flakes, cornmeal mush, polished rice, etc. (brown rice is less acid forming)
All high starch and protein foods (starchy foods in combination with fruits or proteins are acid combinations and should be avoided)

Alkaline-Forming Foods

Most fruits, fresh and dried. Exceptions are large prunes, plums, and cranberries.

Apples	Grapefruit	Pears
Apricots	Lemons	Pineapples
Berries	Limes	Raisins
Dates	Oranges	Small prunes
Figs (unsulphured)	Peaches	

Most vegetables, fresh and dehydrated. Exceptions are legumes (dried beans) and rhubarb.

Asparagus	Honey	Radishes
Beets	Kohlrabi	Rutabaga
Cabbage	Lettuce	Spinach
Carob	Mushrooms	Sprouts
Carrots	Olives (ripe)	String Beans
Cauliflower	Onions	Sweet Potatoes
Celery	Oyster Plant	Tomatoes
Eggplant	Parsnips	Turnips
Green Peas		

Milk, all forms: buttermilk, clabber, sour milk, cottage cheese and cheese

Food Combinations

The Edgar Cayce readings greatly stress the value of observing certain food combinations as well as avoiding the harm caused by others. The digestive chemistry is affected by the combinations of foods we eat. Some combinations are helpful, while others tax the body and interfere with proper assimilation of nutrients. The following extracts from the readings contain the basics of the Cayce philosophy on food combining:

As we find, there is . . . an unbalancing in the alkalinity of the system. Not by the foods themselves; rather the manner of their combination. For, as indicated, there should not be taken starches and sweets at the same meal, or so much together (That's why that ice cream is so much better than pie, for a body!).   340-32

(Q) What foods can be used with fresh citrus fruits to make a complete meal?
(A) Any foods that may be eaten at any time, save whole grain cereals.   2072-14

(Q) Is the quart of milk a day, and orange juice, helpful?
(A) Orange juice and milk are helpful, but these would be taken at opposite ends of the day; not together.   274-9

(Q) What foods should I avoid?
(A) Rather is it the combination of foods that makes for disturbance with most physical bodies, as it would with this. In the activities of the body in its present surroundings, those tending toward the greater alkaline reaction are preferable. Hence avoid combinations where corn, potatoes, rice, spaghetti or the like are taken all at the same meal . . . all of these tend to make for too great a quantity of starch—especially if any meat is taken at such a meal. If no meat is taken, these make quite a difference. For the activities of the gastric flow of the digestive system are the re-

quirements of one reaction in the gastric flow for starch and another for proteins, or for the activities of the carbohydrates as
combined with starches of this nature . . . Then, in the combinations, do not eat great quantities of starch with the proteins or
meats. If sweets and meats are taken at the same meal, these are
preferable to starches. Of course, small quantities of breads with
sweets are all right, but do not have in large quantities. . .

Then, do not combine also the reacting acid fruits with
starches, other than *whole wheat bread!* that is, citrus fruits, oranges, apples, grapefruit, limes or lemons or even tomato juices.
And do not have cereals (which contain the greater quantity of
starch than most) at the same meal with the citrus fruits. 416-9

Most reducing diets do not recommend two starches at the
same meal. Another reason for not filling up with starches is, of
course, that we should not crowd out the leafy green and yellow
vegetables and fruits that we need. The normal diet is one that
nourishes the body properly but does not make it overweight or
underweight.

The readings give us other guidelines on combinations. For
example, lemon or lime juice can be effectively added to other
citrus fruit juices.

It will be much better if you will add a little lime with the orange juice, and a little lemon with the grapefruit—not too much,
but a little. It will be much better and act much better with the
body. For, many of these are hybrids, you see.   3525-1

When orange juice is taken add lime or lemon juice to same;
four parts orange juice to one part lime or lemon.   3823-3

Take plenty of citrous fruit juices . . . With the orange juice put
a little lemon—that is, for a glass of orange juice put about two
squeezes from a good lemon . . . so that there will be at least a
quarter to half a teaspoonful. With the grapefruit juice put a little
lime; about eight to ten drops. Stir these well, of course, before
taking.   2072-3

Mornings—whole grain cereals or citrus fruit juices, though

not at the same meal. When using orange juice, combine lime with it. When using grapefruit juice, combine lemon with it—just a little.   1523-17

Here is another example of food combinations emphasized in the Cayce readings but not found elsewhere: a judicious use of vegetables growing above the ground versus those growing below the ground. The readings give no explanation for this distinction; or perhaps no one asked for it. At any rate, it seems to be an important aspect of the normal diet as well as diets recommended in the readings for various bodily ailments.

> Normal diet . . . Use at least three vegetables that grow above the ground to one that grows under the ground . . .   3373-1

> Have at least one meal each day that includes a quantity of raw vegetables; such as cabbage, lettuce, celery, carrots, onions and the like. Tomatoes may be used in their season.
>
> *Do* have plenty of vegetables above the ground; at least three of these to one below the ground. Have at least one leafy vegetable to every one of the pod vegetables taken.   2602-1

We come finally to the use of fats and butter. Modern dietary guidelines advise against the use of much fat in the diet. The Cayce readings (1901 through 1944) deemphasize the use of fat throughout the diet. Meats are not to be fried; vegetables are not to be cooked with fat meats; the lean portions of meats instead of the fat portions are nearly always suggested; and butter is mentioned as a light seasoning, along with salt, for vegetables.

Vitamins and Minerals

The need for vitamins and minerals is now widely recognized, and much is known about their functions and sources. The readings, however, add a great deal to this knowledge. Vitamins, one reading explains, are "The creative forces working with the body energies for the renewing of the body!" (3511-1) Another explains that they are food for the glands or "that from which the glands take those necessary influences to supply the energies to enable the varied organs of the body to reproduce themselves." (2072-9) The glands, it is further explained, control the supply of materials for rebuilding or reproducing the various tissues in the body, while vitamins are elements or forces that enable each organ to carry on its creative function or generative activity.

The readings supply little-recognized facts concerning functions of various vitamins: for example, vitamin A, in addition to other functions, is important for nerves, bone, and the brain force; vitamin B, in addition to facilitating the functioning of nerves, also supplies "to the chyle that ability for it to control the influence of fats, which is necessary . . . to carry on the reproducing of the oils that prevent the tenseness in the joints, or that prevent the joints from becoming atrophied or dry, or to creak." (2072-9)

The readings also explain that a part of the function of vitamin C is to supply "the necessary influences to the flexes of every nature throughout the body, whether of a muscular or tendon nature, or a heart reaction, or a kidney contraction . . . the batting of the eye, or the supplying of the saliva and the muscular forces in face." (2072-9) A vitamin C deficiency results in "bad eliminations from the incoordination of the excretory functioning of the alimentary canal, as well as the heart, liver and lungs, through the expelling of those forces that are a part of the structural portion of the body." (2072-9)

From the foregoing it would seem that vitamins are even more important than we had realized. We are also told that vitamins are only a combination of basic elements already found in the body, "given a name mostly for confusion . . . by those who would tell you what to do for a price!" (2533-6) We are then warned against taking supplementary vitamins over long periods of time, lest the body, if it comes to rely upon them, cease to produce them in the body, even though the food values are kept in balance. Conversely, there may be an overabundance of vitamins, and unless "activities physical for the body are such as to put same into *activity* they become drosses . . . " (341-31) In such cases these unused vitamins act very much as bacilli and are destructive to tissue, affecting the plasma of the blood supply or the excretory system and lymph.

In most instances the readings agree with accepted dietary opinions as to which foods are rich in vitamins, for example, those that are yellow in color—yellow peaches and apples, squashes, carrots, citrus fruits, etc. However, the readings add some facts not generally recognized:

> Quite a dissertation might be given as to the effect of tomatoes upon the human system. Of all the vegetables, tomatoes carry most of the vitamins in a well-balanced assimilative manner for the activities in the system. Yet if these are not cared for properly, they may become very destructive to a physical organism; that is, if they ripen after being pulled, or if there is the contamination with other influences . . .
> The tomato is one vegetable that in most instances (because of the greater uniform activity) is preferable to be eaten after being canned, for it is then much more uniform.   584-5

The value of gelatin in the diet is recognized, but the reasons for its benefits have puzzled nutritionists, since the amount of energy it supplies is out of proportion to the caloric value of its known elements. The readings give this explanation:

> It isn't the vitamin content [in gelatin] but it is ability to work with the activities of the glands, causing the glands to take from that absorbed or digested the vitamins that would not be active if there is not sufficient gelatin in the body . . . here may be mixed with any chemical that which makes the rest of the system susceptible or able to call from the system that needed. It becomes then, as it were, "sensitive" to conditions. Without it [the gelatin] there is not that sensitivity.   849-75

Methods of preparing food may preserve or destroy much of the vitamin content. Thus fresh foods should, of course, be used as fresh as possible. Frozen vegetables, the readings say, have usually lost "much of the vitamin content . . . unless there is the re-enforcement in same when these are either prepared for food or when frozen." (462-14)

There is the possibility, of course, that this was true only of the slow-freezing methods of that time (1942) and may not hold true with the flash-freezing methods used commercially at present. Fruits, however, lose little of their vitamin content by freezing, according to the readings. Cooking foods quickly by the steam-pressure method, the readings relate, preserves the vitamins, contrary to some nutritional opinions. (See 462-14 and 340-31.) Also recommended is cooking in Patapar paper, a parchment paper, in order to preserve the juices containing much of the vitamin value. (See 1963-2 and 1196-7.) One reading, emphasizing the need for more vitamin B_1, recommended that "all of the vegetables [be] cooked in their *own* juices, and the body eating the juices with same." (2529-1)

The need for certain minerals was given in numerous readings. Often mentioned are calcium, phosphorus, and iron. While all the minerals are undoubtedly of importance, these three were most often found to be insufficient in the diets of those for whom physical readings were given, and we may assume that they are often lacking in the average diet.

> Keep plenty of those foods that supply calcium to the body. These we would find especially in raw carrots, cooked turnips and turnip greens, all characters of salads—especially as of water cress, mustard and the like; these especially taken raw . . .
>
>   1968-6

> When there is a great deal of fowl taken—that is, of chicken, goose, duck, turkey or the like, [chew] the bony pieces or [make] broths of same . . .   808-15

Milk and milk products rich in calcium are highly recommended. One individual was told, "*preferably* the raw milk *if* certified milk!" (275-24) Another reading, given January 17, 1944, for a two-year-old child, warned, however: " . . . raw milk—provided it is from cows that don't eat certain characters of food. If they eat dry food, it is well, if they eat certain types of weeds or grass grown this time of year, it won't be so good for the body." (2752-3)

> The phosphorus forming foods are principally carrots, lettuce (rather the leaf lettuce, which has more soporific activity than

the head lettuce), shell fish, salsify, the *peelings* of Irish potatoes
. . . and things of such natures . . . Citrus fruit juices, plenty of
milk—the Bulgarian [yogurt] the better, or the fresh milk that is
warm with the animal heat which carries more of the phosphorus . . .   560-2

"Let the iron be rather taken in the foods [instead of from me-
dicinal sources], as it is more easily assimilated from the vegetable forces . . . " (1187-9) Foods high in iron are spinach, lentils,
red cabbage, berries, raisins, liver, grapes, pears, onions, and asparagus.

As sources of minerals in general, or in combination these are
given: " . . . cereals that carry the heart of the grain; vegetables of
the leafy kind; fruit and nuts . . . " (1131-2) Rolled or cracked
wheat, not cooked too long, is recommended to "add to the
body the proper proportions of iron, silicon and the vitamins
necessary to build up the blood supply that makes for resistance
in the system." (840-1) And the almond (recommended in several readings to guard against or counteract a tendency toward
cancer) "carries more phosphorus and iron in a combination
easily assimilated than any other nut." (1131-2)

Physiological Effects of Food

In recommending specific foods, the readings attribute to
them certain physiological effects. Some of these may be due to
little-understood effects of the vitamins they contain. Others
apparently have effects aside from vitamin or mineral content.

They [raw green peppers] are better in combination than by
themselves. Their tendency is for an activity to the pylorus; not
the activity in the pylorus itself, but more in the activity from the
flow of the pylorus to the churning effect upon the duodenum in
its digestion. Hence it is an activity for *digestive* forces.

Peppers, then taken with green cabbage, lettuce, are very good
for this body; taken in moderation.   404-6

About beef juice taken in small sips, more than one person
was told the following:

This . . . will work towards producing the gastric flow through the intestinal system, first in the salivary reactions to the very nature of the properties themselves, second with the gastric flow from the upper portion of the stomach or through the cardiac reaction at the end of the esophagus that produces the first of the lacteals' reaction to the gastric flows in the stomach or digestive forces themselves; thirdly making for an activity through the pylorus and the duodenum that becomes stimulating to the activity of the flows without producing the tendencies for accumulation of gases.   1100-10

Meats, especially glandular meats such as calf's liver, brains, and tripe, were advised for their blood-building properties. More often, fish, fowl, and lamb—never fried—were recommended. Fowl should be "prepared in such a way that more of the bone structure itself" is used, according to the readings, not only for the actual calcium content of the bones, but also "that better reaction for the [assimilation of] calcium through the system is obtained . . ." (1523-8) Another reading (5069-1) also stated that "Chewing the bones will be worth more to the body in strengthening and in the eliminations" and added that when these are stewed, the lid should be kept on "so that the boiling will not carry off that which is best to be taken." Cooked long enough in a pressure cooker, the bones dissolve.

Certain vegetables were recommended for their effect in protecting the body against communicable diseases: "Plenty of lettuce should always be eaten by almost *every* body; for this supplies an effluvium in the blood stream itself that is a destructive force to most of those influences that attack the blood stream. It's a purifier." (404-6) Raw vegetables, such as tomatoes, lettuce, celery, spinach, carrots, beet tops, mustard greens, and onions were said to "make for purifying of the *humor* in the lymph blood as this is absorbed by the lacteal ducts as it is digested." (840-1) Cooked onions and beets were also said to be blood purifiers.

Of the fruits, raw apples were recommended as a purifying food: " . . . if raw apples are taken, take them and *nothing* else— three days of raw apples only, and then olive oil, and we will cleanse *all* toxic forces from any system!" (820-2) Raw apples under other circumstances, however, were advised against, unless eaten between meals with no other food. (See 820-2 and 567-7.)

That portion of carrots close to the top "carries the vital energies, stimulating the optic reactions between kidneys and the optics." (3051-6) Potato peelings are said to be "strengthening, carrying those influences . . . that are active with the glands of the system." (820-2) These influences or "vital energies" referred to may also be the vitamins, minerals, or both.

Vegetables, one reading notes, "will build gray matter faster than will meat or sweets!" (900-386)

Jerusalem artichokes were recommended for a number of diabetic individuals with the explanation that the artichokes carry those properties that have an insulin reaction, that will produce a cleansing for the kidneys as well as producing the tendency for the reduction of the excess sugar . . ." (480-39) One individual was also told that artichokes would "tend to correct those inclinations for the incoordination between the activities of the pancreas as related to the kidneys and bladder." (1523-7) This vegetable was never recommended in large amounts, rather one the size of a hen's egg—in some cases once a day, in others once or twice a week, and alternately raw and cooked.

Another physiological effect of foods, and one repeated in many readings, is the effect of eating foods grown in the vicinity where the body resides, rather than those shipped in. This prepares the system to acclimate itself to any given territory." (3542-1) And it "will more quickly adjust a body to any particular area or climate than any other thing." (4047-1) Further, this is more important "than any specific set of fruits, vegetables or what not." (4047-1)

Interestingly, the idea of eating locally grown foods is an important part of the macrobiotic diet, which is based on ancient traditional Chinese medicine. It is also a principle of the Ayurvedic healing philosophy of India. It is believed that this recommendation had to do with eating foods in a seasonal cycle, thus harmonizing our bodies with nature's rhythms.

The "Do Nots"

One individual was advised, "Then, it is well that the body not become as one that couldn't do this, that or the other; or as a slave to an idea of a set diet." (1568-2) Nevertheless, the readings frequently recommended that certain foods and combinations of foods be avoided.

Starches and sweets, except in small amounts, should not be taken at the same meal; nor should there be several starchy foods taken together, since this produces too much acidity in the system. Neither should bread and other starches that grow above the ground be taken with meats. Potatoes, especially the peelings, are preferable to breads consumed with meats.

That citrus fruits should not be taken with cereals was a consistent warning. One reading gave this explanation:

> ... for this *changes* the acidity in the stomach to a detrimental condition; for citrus fruits will act *as* an eliminant when taken alone, but when taken with cereals it becomes as *weight*—rather than as an active force in the gastric forces of the stomach itself.
>
> 481-1

Another common food combination was consistently warned against:

> If coffee is taken, do not take milk in same. If tea is taken, do not take milk in same. This is hard on the digestion ...   5097-1

From the information given in different readings, apparently the effect of coffee or tea alone varies—for some individuals it is harmful; for others it is not.

Onions and radishes (raw) should not be taken at the same meal with celery and lettuce, one individual was told, "though either of these may be taken at different times . . ." (2732-1)

> (Q) What effect has alcohol when you eat raw oysters?
> (A) It produces a chemical reaction that is bad for *most* stomachs. Oysters should never be taken with whiskey.   2853-1

Fried foods should never be eaten, according to the readings, nor vegetables cooked with bacon or fats. Canned foods containing superficial or artificial preservatives should be avoided. Benzoate of soda was specifically mentioned as one of these. Carbonated drinks in most cases were warned against, being referred to as "slop." (5545-2) Cane sugar should not be used in large quantities.

Warning is given against using some foods cooked in aluminum, especially where "a disturbed hepatic eliminating force [exists] . . . " (1196-7) for this "produces a hardship upon the activities of the kidneys as related to the lower hepatic circulation, or [affects] the uric acid that is a part of the activity of the kidneys in eliminating same from the system." (843-7) Specifically mentioned were tomatoes and cabbage: " . . .there are some foods that are affected in their activity by aluminum—especially in the preparation of certain fruits, or tomatoes, or cabbage. But most others, it is very well." (1852-1)

Many readings recommended that bananas not be eaten, unless, like raw apples, they are taken alone, uncombined with other food.

When rabbits are cleaned, "be sure the tendon in both left legs is removed, or that as might cause a fever." (2514-4)

Warnings were repeatedly given against eating pork, except for a little crisp breakfast bacon occasionally. One individual was told of the result, in her case, of eating pork:

> The character of dross it makes in the body-functioning causes a fungi that produces in the system a crystallization of the muscles and nerves in portions of the body . . . These [distresses] began as acute pain, rheumatic or neuritic . . . This is pork—the effect of same.   3599-1

Red meats, or heavy meats not well cooked, were frequently warned against, while fish, fowl, and lamb were recommended, and wild game, properly prepared, was said to be preferable to other meats. (See 2514-4.)

Meat—to Eat or Not to Eat

Whether an individual should eat meat or abstain has long been a disputed question among both health-conscious and spiritually minded individuals. The information in the readings on this subject is consistent:

> Meats of certain characters are necessary in the body-*building* forces in this system, and should not be wholly abstained from in the present. Spiritualize those influences, those activities, rather than abstaining.   295-10

Another reading had this to say:

> This, to be sure, is not an attempt to tell the body to go back to eating meat, but do supply, then, through the body forces, supplements, either in vitamins or in substitutes. [This is necessary] for those who would hold to these [vegetarian] influences—but purifying of mind is of the mind, not of the body. For, as the Master gave, it is not that which entereth in the body, but that which cometh out that causes sin. It is what one does with the purpose, for all things are pure in themselves, and are for the sustenance of man, body, mind, and soul, and remember—these must work together . . .   5401-1

This, too, was given in answer to a question about following a meatless diet:

> . . . this from the material angle is not an absolute necessity—but in all good conscience keep that as thy *soul* (we didn't say *heart*)—thy *soul*—desires.   1554-6

The Cayce normal diet, then, with its abundance of fresh vegetables, fruits, whole grains, and its limited use of meats, is well suited to a vegetarian or other well-balanced healthy diet if that is the soul's desire.

Attitudes and Emotions

What importance do attitudes and emotions have in relation to foods? Much, according to the readings. It is well known that strong emotions such as anger, fear, or worry have an adverse effect upon the digestive system. This is confirmed in the readings to the extent that they advise, *"never,* under strain, when very tired, very excited, very mad, should the body take foods in the system . . ." (137-30)

"The body is the temple of the living God." This idea, told repeatedly in the Bible, is reiterated and enlarged upon throughout the Cayce readings. If we would keep that temple in such a condition as to glorify the Maker, it is imperative that we learn and adhere to certain laws, certain rules in regard to the nutritional needs of the body, for "what we think and what we eat—combined together—*make* what we *are;* physically and mentally." (288-38)

But the readings go further concerning the effect of attitude upon the assimilation of food and what mind "as a builder" accomplishes in constructing the body:

That thou eatest, *see* it *doing* that *thou* would *have* it do. Now there is often considered as to why do those of either the vegetable, mineral, or combination compounds, have different effects under different conditions? It is the *consciousness* of the *individual body!* Give one a dose of clear *water,* with the impression that it will act as salts—how often will it act in that manner?

Just as the impressions to the whole of the organism, for each cell of the blood stream, each corpuscle, is a whole *universe* in itself . . . One that fills the mind, the very being, with an expectancy of God will see His movement, His manifestation, in the wind, the sun, the earth, the flowers, the inhabitant *of* the earth; and so as is builded in the body, is it to gratify *just* an appetite, or is it taken to fulfill an office that *will* the better make, the better magnify, that the body, the mind, the soul, *has* chosen to stand *for?* and it will not matter so much what, where, *when*—but knowing *that* it is consistent with that—that is desired to be accomplished *through* that body!

As has been given of old, when the children of Israel stood

with the sons of the heathen and all ate from the king's table [Daniel 1:5-17], that which was taken that only exercised the imagination of the body in physical desires—as strong drink, strong meats, condiments that magnify desires with the body— this builded as Daniel well understood, not for *God's* service— but he chose rather that the *everyday,* the common things would be given, that the bodies, the minds, might be a more perfect channel for the manifestations of *God;* for the forces of the Creator are in *every* force that is made manifest in the earth. 341-31

May we, as Daniel, choose that which will build such a temple to serve, magnify, and glorify God!

2

Fruits and Vegetables

*T*he readings place the greatest emphasis upon fruits and vegetables—from leafy greens and yellow vegetables to tomatoes and citrus fruits.

Include in the diet often raw vegetables prepared in various ways, not merely as a salad but scraped or grated and combined with gelatin . . .   3445-1

Then the diet: Do have often the raw vegetables such as celery, lettuce, carrots and watercress. Prepare these often . . . with gelatin. Do not throw away the juices when grating or preparing any of these, but include the juices also in the gelatin, for the greater amount of the vitamins necessary.   3413-1

Plenty of raw as well as cooked carrots. Have plenty of lettuce, tomatoes in moderation . . . raw cabbage with same occasionally . . . Not too much of potatoes, but more of the skins. Plenty of onions, raw as well as cooked. Plenty of all forms of the bulbular vegetables—peas, beans . . .   480-52

Have more of the vegetables—the leafy variety would be preferable to those of the bulbular nature or such as beans, peas or the like (that is, the dried, see?)   1657-2

Fruits

Fresh, ripe fruits may be served raw in a variety of combinations as salads and juices, and are so delicious as is that, except for apples, there seems little reason for cooking them. Raw apples were often advised against in the readings and never, to our knowledge, recommended as part of the regular diet, other than in the apple diet:

> . . . three days of raw apples only, and then olive oil [one-half cup], and we will cleanse *all* toxic forces from any system! 820-2

Fully ripe fruits, especially when ripened on the tree or vine, have a greater vitamin content as well as better flavor. Newly picked fruit should be chilled immediately, handled carefully to avoid bruising, washed quickly, and peeled or cut just before using. These methods will ensure a higher level of nutrients. Berries should be washed before being stemmed, rather than after, but should not be washed before storing, as they bruise easily. If it is unavoidable that fruits should stand for some time after being peeled or cut, discoloration and vitamin loss may be lessened by having them chilled before peeling, by mixing cut fruit with a little lemon juice to retard enzyme activity, and by returning them to the refrigerator as quickly as possible. The same precautions apply to the squeezing of orange juice—the juice should be extracted just before being used, but there is less loss of vitamin C if the oranges are chilled before being squeezed and the juice is kept refrigerated in an airtight container.

Stewed Dried Fruit

Dried fruits should be washed quickly and, if soaked, cooked in the water used for soaking. They may be cooked without soaking or may be tenderized by soaking in hot (boiling) water with no further cooking; but with either method, the water or juice should be saved, as it contains many nutrients.

Method #1: Cover fruit with water and bring to a boil. Remove from heat and allow to stand overnight.

Method #2: Bring 2 cups of water to a boil. Add 1 pound of fruit (dried), cover, reduce heat, and simmer until fruit is tender (about 12 to 15 minutes).

Dried fruits contain a large proportion of sugar and usually require no added sweetening. For variety, bits of lemon or orange rind may be added to prunes, apples, pears, or figs during cooking, and small amounts of cloves and cassia buds, or stick cinnamon may be added to prunes, pears, peaches, or apples.

Stewed dried fruits may be served with cereal, sprinkled with ground nuts or grated coconut, or served with cream as a breakfast dish or healthful dessert; stewed or raw dried fruits may be used in cakes, cookies, confections, and puddings. For the latter, see chapter five, "Desserts and Sweets."

Baked Apricots

½ pound dried apricots
1 C. seeded raisins
2 C. water

½ C. honey
Juice of 1 lemon
1 orange, peeled and sliced

Wash apricots, add raisins and water and place in baking dish. Cover and bake at 325° for 2½ hours. Remove from oven, add honey and lemon juice, stir, and chill. Before serving, top with orange slices. Serves 4.

Mummy Food

For those not familiar with the origin of the mummy food recipe: Edgar Cayce had a dream on December 2, 1937, concerning the discovery of ancient Egyptian records during which a mummy came to life and helped translate these records. The mummy gave directions for the preparation of a food that she required (see 294-189 Reports)—thus the name *mummy food*.

Other readings for particular individuals recommended this

same combination. One such reading was as follows:

> And for this especial body, dates, figs (that are dried) cooked
> with a little corn meal (a very little sprinkled in), then this taken
> with milk, should be almost a spiritual food for the body . . .
>
> 275-45

More detailed instructions were given:

> . . . equal portions of black figs or Assyrian figs and Assyrian
> dates—these ground together or cut very fine, and to a pint of
> such a combination put half a handful of corn meal, or crushed
> wheat. These cooked together . . .   275-45

"Half a handful" is an indefinite amount, and the amount of
water is not given; however, the following recipe combination
has been tried and found satisfactory:

Mummy Food

½ C. chopped pitted dates   1 to 1½ C. water
½ C. chopped dried black figs   1 rounded tbs. cornmeal

In a saucepan, combine the dates, figs, water, and cornmeal.
Cook over low heat, stirring frequently, for ten minutes or
longer. Serve with milk or cream. Serves 2 to 4.

Baked Apples

4 large red or yellow apples   1 tbs. butter
⅓ C. chopped raisins   ¼ C. boiling water
⅓ C. chopped nuts   Milk, cream, or yogurt
3 tbs. honey (optional)   (as topping)
1 tsp. cinnamon, nutmeg, or
   grated lemon rind

Wash and core large red or yellow apples, allowing one for each person to be served. Set in baking dish and stuff center of each with a mixture of the chopped raisins, nuts, and honey, if using. Sprinkle with cinnamon, nutmeg, or grated lemon rind. Divide the butter into 4 equal pieces and place on top of each apple. Add ¼ cup boiling water to the baking dish. Cover and bake in 375° oven until tender, about 20 minutes or longer, depending on variety of apples. Serve hot or cold, topped with milk, cream, or yogurt. Serves 4.

Baked Pears

4 medium-sized pears	1 tbs. lemon juice
¼ C. boiling water	2 tsp. butter (optional)
¼ C. honey	

Scrub pears, remove blossom end, and put stem-side-up in baking dish. Mix honey, boiling water, and lemon juice and pour around pears. Add 2 tsp. butter if desired. Cover and bake at 375° for 1 hour, basting occasionally. If large pears are used, they may be cut in half, lengthwise, the cut surface brushed with lemon juice, then cooked as above. Serves 4.

Baked Peaches

4 large peaches	¼ C. water
4 tsp. honey	Cinnamon or cloves
2 tsp. butter	

Cut unpeeled, scrubbed peaches in half and remove seed. Place in baking dish, pour ¼ cup water around them. In center of each peach half, put 1 tsp. or more of honey; top each with ½ tsp. butter and sprinkle lightly with cinnamon or cloves. Cover and bake at 350° until tender, about 15 minutes. Serves 4.

Baked Bananas

4 medium-ripe bananas   4 tsp. honey (optional)
2 tsp. lemon juice

Place peeled bananas in shallow baking dish, sprinkle with lemon juice, and add 1 tsp. honey for each banana, if desired. Bake 10 to 15 minutes at 375°. Serves 4.

Applesauce

2 lb. cooking apples   Ground cinnamon or
Raw sugar or honey, to taste   nutmeg, to taste
½ C. water   Grated lemon or orange rind
                                     (optional)

Bring to boil ½ cup water in saucepan. Wash and quarter the apples but do not peel or core them. Add apples to the saucepan, cover, reduce heat, and steam until soft, about 15 minutes. Press apples through a food mill or colander, chill, and sweeten to taste with raw sugar or honey. Flavor with cinnamon or nutmeg, and grated lemon or orange rind, if desired. Serves 4.

Stewed Whole Apples

4 large apples   ½ tsp. cinnamon or nutmeg
1 C. boiling water   ,   2 tsp. butter
2 tsp. raw sugar

Peel washed and cored apples ¼ of the way down and put peeled-side-down in saucepan containing 1 cup boiling water. Cover and boil for 1 minute, then reduce heat and simmer until tender when tested with a toothpick. Turn peeled-side-up, sprinkle with raw sugar and cinnamon or nutmeg, and top with butter. Brown under broiler. Serves 4.

Orange-Apricot Cooler

⅔ C. orange juice   Fresh mint, for garnish
⅓ C. apricot juice or thin purée

Combine the orange juice and apricot juice or purée in a serving glass. Stir to combine and garnish with sprig of fresh mint. Serve cold. Serves 1.

Black Raspberry-Peach Compote

⅓ C. black raspberries   ⅓ C. diced yellow peaches
⅓ C. unsweetened pineapple juice

Combine raspberries, pineapple juice, and peaches in a small bowl. Chill in refrigerator until serving time. Serves 1.

Pear-Persimmon Compote

1 medium fresh pear,   2 large unpeeled California
   washed, unpeeled   persimmons, frozen
1⅓ C. pineapple or grapefruit juice

Dice pear and soak in juice for ½ hour. Just before serving, cut frozen persimmons into small cubes and combine with the pears and juice. Serves 4.

Decorative Juice Cubes

Use any clear, light-colored juice. Half fill ice cube trays with juice and set into freezing compartment until ice crystals form over top. Quickly arrange small, fresh raspberries, strawberries, or bits of orange or lemon peel with small mint leaves, to simulate flower arrangement, in center of each cube. Freeze until solid, then add enough juice to fill the tray and complete freezing. Add these cubes to glasses of chilled juice just before serving.

Frozen Fruit Purées

Beat or mash through colander or food mill soft stewed apricots, plums, peaches, or other fruit. Add honey to taste. Freeze in freezing compartment, stirring or beating 2 or 3 times. May be served in sherbet glasses with meat course or as dessert, or stored in freezer in plastic containers for use when fresh fruit is not available.

Fruit Aspics

½ C. fruit juice
1 tbs. gelatin

1½ C. puréed fruit
1 tbs. lemon juice (optional)

In a saucepan, combine the fruit juice and gelatin, and soak for 5 minutes. Heat slowly until gelatin is dissolved and add the puréed fruit. If the purée is not tart, add lemon juice. Pour the mixture into the mold and chill until firm. Unmold and serve with meat. Serves 4.

Sunny Compote

2 large ripe bananas

½ tsp. lemon juice

1 C. plump, moist figs   ¼ C. chopped sunflower seeds

Slice bananas and figs and place in a bowl with the lemon juice, tossing together to combine. Sprinkle the chopped sunflower seeds over the fruit and tightly cover the bowl until serving time. Serves 4.

Berry Bowl

1 C. fresh strawberries   1 C. black cherries
1 C. black raspberries   2 tbs. honey (optional)
1 C. raw blueberries   2 tbs. chopped nuts or sun
                                   flower seeds (optional)

Combine the berries in a bowl and keep covered until serving time. Add honey and nuts or sunflower seeds, if desired. Serves 4.

Raw Winter Pears

4 ripe winter pears   ¼ tsp. powdered ginger
2 tbs. honey or maple syrup

Pare, core, and slice pears and place in a serving dish. Drizzle with honey or maple syrup and season with ginger. Cover until serving time. Serves 4.

Apricot Conserve

1 lb. ripe fresh apricots   Blanched ground almonds,
Honey, to taste   as needed

Pit and mash the apricots and place in a bowl. Stir in the desired amount of honey and thicken with blanched ground almonds. Serves 4.

Strawberry Sherbet

1 pkg. frozen strawberries   1 C. water
1 C. orange juice   Whipped cream, optional

Mash strawberries, add orange juice and water. Pour into refrigerator tray and freeze. Serve with heavy whipped cream, if desired. Serves 4 to 6.

Fresh Peach Mousse

5 peaches, fresh or dried   2 tbs. maple syrup
½ pt. whipped cream   ⅓ C. ground almonds

Place either fresh peaches or soaked dried peaches in a food processor and purée. Transfer to a bowl and chill in the refrigerator. Fold in the whipped cream. Add maple syrup and nuts. Chill again before serving. Serves 4 to 6.

Banana Delight

2 C. dried figs, stemmed   ¼ C. chopped English
    and finely chopped   walnuts or peanuts
4 bananas

Place chopped figs in a bowl and cover with hot water. Cover bowl and let stand overnight or several hours. Purée figs in a food processor and reserve. Slice the bananas and place in a serving bowl. Pour the mashed figs over the bananas and sprinkle with walnuts or peanuts. Keep covered, unchilled, until serving time. Serves 4 to 6.

Vegetables

If eighty percent of our food is to be alkaline producing, as the Cayce readings recommend, then at least fifty percent will probably be in the form of vegetables. Certainly it is worthwhile to use considerable care in their selection and preparation.

Vegetables should be freshly gathered, if possible. Frozen vegetables, however, are preferable to those that have been several days in shipment, or to commercially canned foods, which have added chemical preservatives.

Bright yellow and intensely green vegetables provide the greatest concentration of minerals and vitamins. Green leafy vegetables are also rich in iron and calcium. Perhaps this is why the readings advised at least one leafy vegetable with each one of the pod variety.

Nutritive value is lost by peeling, since most of the minerals are concentrated just under the skin; by boiling, which leaches out the minerals, sugars, and water-soluble vitamins; and by exposing the vegetable to oxygen and light, which causes enzymes to destroy the vitamins.

Vegetables, except for potatoes and dry onions, should be washed, dried, and returned to the refrigerator. When cooked, they should be heated rapidly, as enzymes—inactive when cold—are killed by heat. Having the cooking pots heated and filled with steam, plus leaving the lid on during cooking, are important, as vitamin B is destroyed by heating in the presence of light. Alkali destroys vitamin C; thus, soda should never be used in cooking vegetables. Minerals in hard water are another offender in this respect. Contact with copper or iron also destroys vitamin C and should be carefully avoided.

Cooking vegetables by the steam-pressure method helps to retain the vitamins, as the readings point out (462-14), but care must be taken to avoid overcooking when using this method. Cooking time should be checked precisely and the pot cooled immediately when cooking time has expired.

Cooking in Patapar paper (trade name of Paterson Parchment Co., Bristol, Pa.) was recommended in the readings (1196-

6). This type of cooking parchment and other varieties are usually available in health food stores or specialty food shops. Cooking in parchment paper preserves nutrients, retains the juices of the vegetable (which contain the vitamins and minerals), and excludes oxygen and light. The paper should be tied tightly around the vegetable to eliminate air pockets and placed into rapidly boiling water. Timetables must be relied on to indicate when sufficiently cooked.

Timetable for Steaming Vegetables

	Minutes		Minutes
Artichokes, Globe	20-30	Garbanzo beans	180
Artichokes, Jerusalem	6-10	Kale	8-10
Asparagus	8-10	Kohlrabi	9-10
Beans, fresh limas	15-20	Leek, sliced	8-10
Beans, green or wax	15-20	Mushrooms, chopped	5-8
Beet leaves	3-5	Mustard greens, shredded	5-8
Beets, grated	5-8	Okra	5-8
Beets, whole small	30-35	Onions, sliced	5-8
Broccoli	8-10	Onions, whole	20-25
Brussels sprouts	10-12	Parsley	5
Cabbage, Chinese	4-7	Parsnips, sliced	10-15
Cabbage, quartered	4-7	Parsnips, whole	20
Cabbage, shredded	3	Peas, fresh green	8-10
Carrots, grated	5-8	Potatoes, halved sweet	30-35
Carrots, small whole	20-25	Potatoes, halved white	30-35
Cauliflower, in pieces	8-10	Rutabagas, cubed	25-30
Celery	8-10	Spinach	3-5
Celery root	20-25	Squash, summer	8
Corn, fresh	3-5	Swiss chard	8
Dandelion greens	3-5	Turnip greens, shredded	5
Eggplant, cubed	8-10	Turnips	20-25
Endive	3-5	Tomatoes	3-5

Lemon Broccoli

1½ lb. broccoli   2 tbs. honey

1 tbs. lemon juice

Trim outer leaves and tough ends of broccoli, split any thick stalks, then cut stalks and flowerets into 3-inch lengths. Steam, covered, in a small amount of salted water in a medium saucepan for 10 minutes or just until crisp-tender. Drain carefully, retaining water, and spoon into heated serving bowl. Mix lemon juice, water drained from broccoli, and honey. Drizzle over broccoli. Serves 4 to 6.

Steamed Celery Cabbage

1 medium head Chinese cabbage   1 tsp. celery seeds
1 tsp. salt

Shred cabbage fine, wash well, and drain. Place in a large frying pan (no need to add water), sprinkle with salt and celery seeds, and cover. Steam 3 minutes or just until crisp-tender. Serve with cooking juices. Serves 4 to 6.

Asparagus with Citrus Sauce

1½ lb. asparagus, steamed   Dash of salt
2 tbs. butter   Grated rind of ½ orange
2 egg yolks, well beaten   1 tbs. lemon juice
½ tsp. paprika   4 tbs. orange juice

Set steamed asparagus aside. To make sauce, combine butter, egg yolks, paprika, salt, and grated orange rind. Cook over hot water, stirring constantly until thick and smooth. Add orange juice and lemon juice and beat until smooth. Serve over asparagus. Serves 4 to 6.

Sliced Baked Beets

In this and other recipes, celery may be substituted for onions, if desired.

8 small beets, sliced	1½ tbs. butter
1 tbs. honey	1⅛ tsp. lemon juice
⅜ tsp. salt	2½ tbs. water
⅛ tsp. nutmeg	1 small onion, chopped

Place beets in layers in greased baking dish. Season with honey, salt, and nutmeg. Dot with butter, add lemon juice, water, and onion. Bake covered in a 350° oven for 30 minutes, or until tender. Sprinkle with parsley and serve. Serves 4 to 5.

Baked Acorn Squash with Pineapple

3 acorn squashes, halved	½ C. unsweetened crushed
½ C. butter	pineapple, drained
¼ C. honey	¼ tsp. ground nutmeg
	1 tsp. salt

Place cleaned squash halves in a greased baking dish and divide 2 tbs. of the honey and 4 tbs. of the butter equally into the center of each half. Cover and bake at 400° for 30 minutes or until tender. Scoop cooked squash out of shells, leaving about ¼ inch remaining in shells. Mash the cooked squash and set aside. In a small saucepan combine the remaining 4 tbs. butter and 2 tbs. honey with the pineapple, nutmeg, and salt, heating and stirring until well blended. Combine with mashed squash and mix well. Spoon the squash mixture back into shells and return to a hot oven for 15 minutes. Serves 6.

Baked Carrots

1 lb. coarsely shredded carrots
¼ C. minced onions
¼ C. water

2 tbs. butter
1 tsp. salt
¼ tsp. celery salt

Combine all ingredients in a lightly oiled baking dish. Cover and bake at 375° for 45 minutes or until tender. Serves 4.

Green Peas with Celery and Ripe Olives

2 tbs. vegetable oil
2 C. sliced celery, cut in 2-inch
   diagonal pieces
2 pkg. frozen peas, partly thawed

20 pitted ripe olives, halved
½ tsp. salt
¼ tsp. pepper
1 tbs. water, if needed

Heat oil in a large frying pan over low heat. Stir the celery into the pan, until celery pieces are coated with oil. Cover and cook celery in oil for 10 minutes, shaking occasionally. Add the peas, cover, and continue cooking over low heat for 6 minutes, shaking several times. Add 1 tbs. water during cooking, if necessary. Stir in olives, salt, and pepper. Serves 6 to 8.

Raw Carrots and Peas

2 C. raw peas

2 C. raw baby carrots

Top and wash baby carrots. Cut them into chunks not much larger than the peas and put both in a covered dish. Serve raw. Neither dressing nor seasoning is needed. They are delicious as is. Serves 4.

Garbanzos Creole

2 C. cooked garbanzos   ½ Spanish onion, chopped
1 C. canned tomatoes   ¼ tsp. honey (optional)

Combine the garbanzos, tomatoes, and onion in a saucepan and simmer covered over low heat until the onion is tender. Honey may be added, if desired. Serve hot. Serves 4.

Succotash

1 pkg. frozen sweet corn   1 tbs. salad oil
1 pkg. frozen green lima beans   ¼ tsp. dried marjoram
   (or home-canned ones)   ¼ C. chopped green
¼ tsp. powdered sea kelp   peppers, for garnish
Pinch of black pepper

Combine the corn and lima beans in a saucepan and simmer together over low heat in a small amount of water, seasoned with sea kelp, dried marjoram, and the salad oil. Add black pepper and garnish with chopped green peppers. Serve hot. Serves 6.

Young Beets and Greens

1 lb. young beets, including greens   1 tbs. honey
4 tbs. salad oil   Dash of cinnamon
2 tbs. cider vinegar

Wash and cook young beets gently until tender, about 10 minutes. Top the beets and peel them. Chop the beet tops and place in a serving dish, with the young beets nested in the center. Dress with oil, vinegar, honey, and a faint dusting of cinnamon. Serves 4.

Jerusalem Artichokes

Jerusalem artichokes, frequently recommended in the readings for individuals with diabetes or a tendency for it, were also said to "produce a cleansing for the kidneys" (480-39) and "to correct those inclinations for the incoordination between the activities of the pancreas as related to the kidneys and bladder." (1523-7) There is no indication whether they are advisable in the normal diet, but they have been used by many as a vegetable rather than as a medicine with no apparent negative effects.

The Jerusalem artichoke, or "starchless potato," is a nutty-flavored tuber containing inulin (not insulin) and levulose, and good amounts of potassium and thiamine. They are good steamed (in Patapar paper, the readings advised) or raw, in salads, grated or thinly sliced. They are planted like potatoes, yield better than potatoes, and are handled and harvested in the same way, except that they are perennials and require a permanent growing space. Also, they will not keep well for any length of time out of the ground, so should be left in the ground under a heavy mulch during the winter and dug up as needed. The blossoms, similar to small sunflowers, reach a height of from six to twelve feet.

Seed Sprouts

This section on sprouts is included not because of specific recommendations in the readings, but because they offer an excellent way of obtaining a fresh supply of alkaline-producing vegetables with all the vitamins and minerals.

In many sections of the country it is difficult to obtain fresh salad greens or vegetables during a long part of the year, and impossible in most areas to have them year-round, "grown in the area where the body is residing . . ." (257-236)

Sprouting seeds increases their vitamin content and changes their starch into a simple sugar, easy to digest. The cooking time of beans, such as navy beans, red beans, etc., which ordinarily require two to three hours, may be shortened to 10 to 15 minutes by sprouting, giving the double advantage of saving fuel and avoiding the destruction of food values that takes place during long cooking.

Many different seeds may be used. Almost every kind of bean—especially mung beans and soybeans—peas, lentils, wheat, rye, oats, corn, barley, millet, alfalfa, clover, and parsley are among those that produce tasty and nutritious sprouts.

As soon as the sprout is seen, it is ready to eat, and the vitamin content continues to increase as the sprout grows. However, many kinds of sprouts become less tasty if allowed to grow too long.

The following is a good rule of thumb

Wheat sprouts—length of the seed
Mung bean sprouts—1½ to 2 inches
Alfalfa sprouts—1 to 2 inches
Pea and soybean sprouts—good either short or long
Lentil sprouts—1 inch
Sunflower seed sprouts—length of seed

How to Sprout Seeds

There are several methods of sprouting seeds. You may have to experiment to find the method that suits you best, but the principle of all methods is the same: the seeds require warmth, moisture, oxygen, and darkness. Seed size often determines which method to use.

Soybean method: Put soybeans in an earthenware pot with the hole in the bottom covered by a piece of crockery. For ¼ pound of beans use a two-quart pot. Pour water over them and drain well. Keep beans warm and moist, sprinkling them with water twice each day (more often if necessary). An optional step is to soak the beans for six hours before placing them in the pot.

Wheat method: Wash wheat, soak overnight, drain and rinse in the morning, add fresh water, and put in a dark place. Repeat draining and rinsing three times a day for three days. On the evening of the third day, drain wheat thoroughly and put in a shallow pan in a dark place until morning, when sprouts should be of the proper length.

Alfalfa method: Place about one tablespoon of alfalfa seed in a wide-mouth jar and cover with water; place a piece of nylon stocking or fine nylon net over the mouth of the jar and secure with a rubber band. Let stand overnight or eight hours, out of light. When time is complete, drain well, rinse slowly and easily, and place jar on its side out of light. At least three times a day, cover with water and drain again. After each draining, return the jar to its side. If the humidity is low, there is danger of the seeds drying out. To avoid this, sprinkle them occasionally throughout the day with water. In three to five days the sprouts will reach a length of one to two inches and be ready for use. Remove the sprouts from the jar, place in large bowl, and rinse carefully to remove the brown hulls, using a colander.

Small seed method: Scatter seed on damp bath towel. Roll towel loosely; sprinkle towel whenever necessary to keep damp. (This method may be most successful with small seeds.)

When sprouts are of the desired length, put in large bowl, wash thoroughly to remove hulls, if necessary, and store in refrigerator in crisper or plastic bag.

Using Sprouts

Sprouts are good by themselves with your favorite seasoning, in sandwiches, salads, or in many cooked dishes. Sprouted wheat added to bread dough makes an interesting variation. Soybean and mung bean sprouts may be served as a cooked vegetable.

Mushroom Chop Suey

Chinese chestnuts and bamboo sprouts are optional ingredients of this recipe, if available. If raw Chinese chestnuts are used, slice thin and add with sauce. Serve with cooked brown rice.

2 tbs. vegetable oil
3 C. onion, diced
3 C. celery, diced
1 C. beef stock or chicken broth
1 can mushrooms, broken or sliced

2 tbs. cornstarch
2 tbs. soy sauce
2 tsp. molasses
1 tsp. salt
1 lb. mung bean or soybean
   sprouts

Heat oil in a skillet over low heat. Add the onion and celery and cook, covered, for 5 minutes. Remove cover, add ¾ cup of the stock or broth and simmer for 10 minutes longer, then add the mushrooms. Mix remaining broth with cornstarch, soy sauce, molasses, and salt. Add to vegetables and cook, stirring constantly until thickened. Add bean sprouts and simmer 5 minutes. Serves 6 to 8.

Chicken and Bean Sprout Chop Suey

2 tbs. butter
½ C. sliced onion
2 C. diced chicken or turkey
1 C. celery, diced
1 can sliced water chestnuts
½ C. chicken bouillon or turkey broth

2 tbs. arrowroot (or cornstarch)
¼ C. water
2 tbs. soy sauce
Salt and pepper, to taste
1 lb. bean sprouts
½ C. slivered almonds

Melt butter in a large skillet over medium-low heat. Add onions, cover, and cook until tender but not brown, about 5 minutes. Remove cover, add chicken or turkey, celery, water chestnuts, broth, and heat to boiling point. Combine arrowroot, water, soy sauce, salt, and pepper. Stir into mixture and cook until thickened. Add sprouts and almonds. Serves 8.

Egg Foo Yung

2 medium onions, finely chopped
3 medium green peppers,
    finely chopped
4 eggs, beaten

2 tbs. vegetable oil
½ tsp. salt
1 lb. fresh bean sprouts

In a bowl, combine the onions, peppers, eggs, oil, salt, and bean sprouts, and mix well. Working in batches, spoon mixture onto a hot oiled grill and sauté until light brown on both sides. Serves 4 to 6.

Soybean Sprout Omelet

A blended vegetable salt, such as Spike, may be used to replace salt in most recipes, if desired.

1 egg, separated
1 tbs. water
1 tsp. salt

2 tbs. soybean sprouts
1 tsp. butter

Beat egg white until frothy. Add water and salt. Continue beating until stiff, then fold in the well-beaten yolk and the bean sprouts. Pour into a hot, buttered omelet pan and cook for 2 minutes over medium heat. Bake in moderate 350° oven for 2 minutes or until done. Serves 1.

Bean Sprout Omelet

3 eggs
1 C. bean sprouts, cooked
½ C. sweet cream

Salt
Sliced radishes, as garnish

Beat eggs until light, add bean sprouts, cream, and salt. Cook in double boiler until eggs are set. Garnish with thin slices of crisp red radishes. Serves 2 to 3.

Mung Bean Sprouts

1 tbs. butter   2 C. mung bean sprouts
½ C. onion, chopped

Heat butter in a skillet over medium heat. Add onions and cook until softened, about 5 minutes. Remove from heat and add mung beans. Shake or carefully stir the mixture until sprouts are well covered with butter and onions. Serves 2.

Alfalfa Sprouts Rarebit

Bragg's Liquid Aminos is an all-purpose seasoning available at natural food stores. It contains all the essential amino acids and tastes similar to soy sauce.

2 C. water   ⅜ C. sesame tahini or
3 tbs. raw cashews   raw nut butter
1 tsp. salt   2 tsp. Bragg's Liquid Aminos
1 tbs. whole wheat pastry flour   (optional)
1 tsp. onion powder   1½ C. alfalfa sprouts
3 tbs. arrowroot powder   4 slices whole wheat toast
                                                Pimento strips and ripe olives,
                                                  as garnish

In a blender, combine the water, cashews, salt, flour, onion powder, and arrowroot and blend well. Pour the mixture into a pan over low heat, and stir constantly until sauce thickens. Remove from heat and add the tahini and aminos, if using, and mix well. Stir in the alfalfa sprouts and serve over whole wheat toast. Garnish with pimento strips and ripe olives. Serves 2.

Salads

Of all the diet recommendations in the Cayce readings, one of the most unvarying is the raw, fresh vegetable salad for the noon meal. Sometimes it was recommended that fruit salads be alternated with these (935-1). Frequently, individuals were advised to prepare raw vegetables with gelatin (3429-1). Some were told not to use any acetic acid or synthetic vinegar with them. Oil dressings, such as olive oil with paprika and the yolk of a hard-boiled egg, were frequently recommended.

Most nutritionists agree on the value of an abundance of raw fresh vegetables, with deep green leaves being rich in vitamins A, C, E, K, P, B_2, folic acid, eight or more B vitamins, iron, copper, magnesium, calcium, and other minerals.

Fresh salad greens should be the basis for most salads, according to the Cayce readings. There are many types of salad greens, each with its own taste and texture, and you may enhance a salad by using a combination of greens along with other salad ingredients. Greens used raw for salads include the following: kale, spinach, dandelion greens, field salad, watercress, Boston lettuce, sour grass, turnip greens, beet greens, finocchi, iceberg lettuce, mustard greens, nasturtium leaves, green cabbage, fresh endive, chicory, bibb lettuce, savoy cabbage, escarole, celery, romaine, and leaf lettuce.

Eggplant Salad

1 medium eggplant
1 medium onion, grated
Juice of one onion

2 tbs. salad oil
2 tbs. minced parsley

Place the whole eggplant in a glass baking dish and bake in a 350° oven for 30 to 45 minutes. Allow to cool. Peel eggplant and cut into cubes. Transfer to a serving bowl and combine with the remaining ingredients. Cover and chill thoroughly in refrigerator before serving. Serves 4.

Jerusalem Artichoke Salad

2 C. cubed Jerusalem artichokes
1 small onion, minced
2 tbs. minced fresh parsley

2 C. shredded romaine
   lettuce
Salad dressing (optional)

Finely chop the artichokes and combine in a bowl with the onion and parsley. Divide romaine onto two salad plates, top with the artichoke mixture, evenly divided. Drizzle with salad dressing, if desired. Serves 2.

Lettuce and Watercress Salad

2 C. shredded lettuce
1 C. watercress

⅔ C. nut meats (walnuts,
   pecans, almonds)
¼ C. lemon juice

Combine watercress and lettuce in a bowl and set aside. Toss nut meats in lemon juice and sprinkle over salad. Serves 2.

Green and Gold Vegetable Bowl

1 lb. cut green beans, cooked
   and drained
1 C. sliced celery
2 lb. sliced carrots, cooked
   and drained
¼ C. salad oil
2 tbs. lemon juice

1 tsp. minced onion
1 tsp. dried parsley flakes
1 tsp. brown sugar
½ tsp. salt
1 small head romaine lettuce
Mayonnaise or salad
   dressing (optional)

Toss beans with celery in small bowl and place carrots in a second bowl. Mix salad oil, lemon juice, onion, parsley flakes, sugar, and salt in a small bowl and drizzle half over carrots and remaining half over beans. Toss each lightly and chill in the refrigerator. Spoon carrot and bean mixture in separate piles in a shallow serving bowl lined with lettuce leaves. Serve with mayonnaise or salad dressing, as desired. Serves 8.

Riviera Green Beans

4 C. torn salad greens
¼ C. minced fresh herbs
2 C. tender green beans,
   cut in 1-inch lengths
1 tbs. green onions, chopped
1 young carrot, sliced thin on a grater

1 C. tiny red or yellow
   vine-ripened tomatoes
½ C. shelled peas
Salad dressing, as desired
Rose hips and paprika, for
   garnish

Place the salad greens in a serving bowl and sprinkle with the fresh herbs. In a separate bowl combine the green beans, onions, carrot, tomatoes, and peas, and toss with a favorite salad dressing. Spoon vegetable mixture over the salad greens. Garnish with rose hips and paprika. Keep covered in refrigerator until serving time. Serves 4.

Raw Vegetable Salad

1 bunch spinach, chopped
2 green onions, chopped
4 sprigs watercress, chopped
1 small cucumber, peeled, seeded,
   and chopped

1 vine-ripened tomato, diced
1 carrot, grated
Mayonnaise or salad dressing,
   to taste
Radish roses, as garnish

In a bowl, combine the spinach, onions, watercress, cucumber, tomato, and carrot. Add mayonnaise or salad dressing to taste and mix well. Garnish with radish roses and serve. Serves 4 to 6.

Cooked Vegetable Salad

1 C. string beans, cooked
1 C. carrots, cooked and cut in strips
1 C. lima beans, cooked
1 C. peas, cooked

⅓ C. salad oil
¼ C. lemon juice
3 tbs. honey
Ripe olives, for garnish

Cut the string beans through the center, lengthwise. Place the green beans, carrots, lima beans, and peas in a bowl and set aside. In a small bowl, combine the oil, lemon juice, and honey until well combined. Pour the lemon-honey dressing over the vegetables and toss gently until well combined. Divide vegetables among individual salad bowls and garnish with ripe olives. Serves 4 to 6.

Crisp Alfalfa Sprout Toss

2 C. minced celery
1 C. alfalfa sprouts
1 C. raisins

2 carrots, grated
¾ C. yogurt or sour cream

In a bowl, combine the celery, alfalfa sprouts, raisins, and carrots, and mix thoroughly. When ready to serve, top salad with yogurt or sour cream. Serves 4 to 6.

Bean Sprout Tomato Salad

1 small head romaine lettuce
2 C. bean sprouts
1 cucumber, thinly sliced
3 vine-ripened tomatoes, thinly sliced

Radishes, for garnish
Ripe olives, for garnish
Sour Cream Dressing
  (see page 61)

Line salad plates with lettuce leaves. Place a layer of bean sprouts on the leaves. Place alternate layers of cucumber and tomato slices over the sprouts, tapering up to a peak. Garnish with ripe olives and radishes. Serve with sour cream dressing. Serves 4 to 6.

Refreshing Alfalfa Sprout Slaw

¾ C. unsweetened crushed
   pineapple, undrained

3 C. chopped cabbage
1 C. alfalfa sprouts

In a bowl, combine the pineapple with its juice, the cabbage, and the sprouts, and mix well. Serves 4 to 6.

Alfalfa Sprout Salad

1 small head romaine lettuce
2 C. alfalfa sprouts
¾ C. cubed avocado
1 C. sliced okra

¾ C. cooked green soybeans
2 small vine-ripened tomatoes,
   sliced
Salad dressing of choice

Line salad plates with lettuce leaves and set aside. In a bowl, combine the sprouts, avocado, okra, and soybeans and mix well. Place the mixture on the lettuce, dividing evenly. Top with tomato slices. Serve with a favorite salad dressing. Serves 4 to 6.

Basic Recipe
for Vegetable Salad Gelatin

1 tbs. gelatin
½ C. cold water
1 C. boiling water or light-colored stock
2 to 4 tbs. honey

1 tbs. grated onion (optional)
2 C. diced vegetables,
   cooked or raw
Boston lettuce leaves

¼ tsp. salt, if water is used   Mayonnaise or yogurt, as
¼ C. lemon juice   garnish

Soak gelatin in cold water and dissolve thoroughly in boiling water or stock. Add honey, salt, lemon juice, and onion, if desired. Chill. When nearly set, add vegetables and chill until firmly set. Line salad plates with lettuce leaves, top with vegetable salad, and garnish with a dollop of mayonnaise or yogurt. Serves 4 to 6.

Gelatin and Alfalfa Sprout Salad

4 tbs. unflavored gelatin   1 C. chopped alfalfa sprouts
½ C. warm water   ¾ C. diced avocado
1½ C. pineapple juice   ¾ C. unsweetened crushed
2 tbs. honey   pineapple, drained
                                     Mayonnaise, as garnish

Soften gelatin in the warm water for 5 minutes. Liquefy with 1 cup of the unsweetened pineapple juice. Cook for few minutes, until gelatin is completely dissolved. Add remaining pineapple juice and honey. Let stand a few minutes, add sprouts, avocado, and pineapple. Pour into mold, chill, and serve topped with mayonnaise. Serves 4 to 6.

Alfalfa Sprout Gelatin Salad

1 envelope unflavored gelatin   1 C. finely shredded cabbage
½ C. cold water   1 C. minced celery
Juice of 1 lemon   ¼ C. chopped green pepper
2 C. boiling water   1 C. alfalfa sprouts
½ C. honey   Romaine lettuce leaves
½ tsp. salt

Soak gelatin in cold water for 5 minutes. Add lemon juice,

boiling water, honey, and salt. Pour into mold. When gelatin begins to set, add cabbage, celery, pepper, and sprouts. When firmly set, cut into wedges and serve on lettuce leaves. Serves 4 to 6.

Alfalfa Sprout and Vegetable Gelatin Salad

1 envelope unflavored gelatin	1 C. shredded carrots
½ C. cold water	½ C. chopped green pepper
Juice of 1 lemon	½ C. thinly sliced cucumber
2 C. boiling water	½ C. thinly sliced radishes
½ C. honey	1 C. alfalfa sprouts
1 tsp. salt	2 C. shredded lettuce

Soak gelatin in cold water for 5 minutes. Add lemon juice, boiling water, honey, and salt. Pour into mold. When gelatin begins to set, add carrots, pepper, cucumber, radishes, and sprouts. Chill. Serve on lettuce. Serves 4 to 6.

Fresh Vegetable Gelatin Salad

2 envelopes unflavored gelatin	1½ C. shredded cabbage
½ C. cold water	¾ C. diced celery
2 C. hot water	¾ C. shredded carrots
⅓ C. honey	¼ C. chopped green pepper
1¼ tsp. salt	2 tbs. diced pimento
¼ C. lemon juice	Shredded crisp greens
⅔ C. ripe olives, pitted and diced	Mayonnaise or yogurt, for garnish

Soften gelatin in cold water, add hot water and stir until dissolved. Stir in honey, salt, and lemon juice. Add olives, cabbage, celery, carrots, green pepper, and pimento, and mix well. Pour into 1¼-quart ring mold or an 8″ x 8″ x 2″ cake pan. Chill until firm. Cut into wedges or squares. Garnish with crisp greens and serve with mayonnaise or yogurt. Serves 8 to 10.

Fresh Fruit Salad or Dessert

Use all your favorite fresh fruits (except pineapple and apples) with unflavored gelatin, for delicious flavor.

1 envelope unflavored gelatin	1 C. hot water
¼ C. cold water	½ C. grapefruit juice
¼ C. honey	1 tbs. lemon juice
⅛ tsp. salt	Fresh fruit, cut up

Soften gelatin in cold water and add honey, salt, and hot water. Stir until dissolved. Add grapefruit and lemon juice. Mix well. Pour 1 cup mixture into mold that has been rinsed in cold water. When mixture begins to thicken, arrange fruit in it. Chill remaining gelatin until it begins to thicken, then whip until frothy and thick and pour on the gelatin mixture. Chill until firm. Serves 6.

Gelatin Fruit Salad

1 envelope unflavored gelatin	¼ C. chopped banana
½ C. boiling water	¼ C. unsweetened crushed
1½ C. unsweetened	pineapple, drained
pineapple juice	2 tbs. chopped orange
1 tbs. lemon juice	2 tbs. finely grated coconut

Dissolve gelatin in boiling water. Place on stove and let boil for 1 minute, stirring constantly. Add pineapple juice and lemon juice. Set aside to cool. When mixture is half set, add the banana, pineapple, orange, and coconut. Pour into individual molds and allow to set, approximately 20 minutes. Serves 4.

Tomato Aspic

4 pkg. unflavored gelatin
2 C. cold tomato juice
5 C. hot tomato juice
1 tsp. salt

¼ tsp. Tabasco
4 tbs. lemon juice
Salad greens
Salad dressing (optional)

Soften gelatin in cold tomato juice. Dissolve thoroughly in very hot tomato juice, stirring well. Season with salt, Tabasco, and lemon juice. Pour into individual molds. When set, unmold on salad greens. Serve plain or with salad dressing. Serves 12.

Tomato-Shrimp Aspic

2 pkg. unflavored gelatin
½ C. cold water
2 C. tomato juice
3 tsp. lemon juice

Salt and pepper, to taste
1 C. celery, chopped
½ C. green olives, chopped
½ C. shrimp

Sprinkle gelatin in cold water to soften. Place over very low heat and stir until dissolved. Remove from heat and stir in tomato juice, lemon juice, salt, and pepper. Chill mixture to unbeaten egg-white consistency. Fold in celery, olives, and shrimp. Turn into a 6-cup mold. Serves 4.

Shrimp Tossed Salad

¼ C. salad oil
1½ tbs. lemon juice
1 tsp. salt
⅛ tsp. pepper
⅛ tsp. dry mustard
⅛ tsp. celery seeds

¼ tsp. grated onion
½ C. sliced ripe olives
1 medium vine-ripened
   tomato, diced
1 C. cleaned, cooked fresh
   shrimp, crab meat, or lobster
4 C. shredded crisp lettuce

In a bowl, combine the oil, lemon juice, salt, pepper, mustard, celery seeds, and onion. Mix well with a fork and reserve. In a salad bowl, place the olives, tomato, seafood, and lettuce. Add the reserved dressing and toss gently to combine. Serves 4 to 6.

Tuna Fish Gelatin Salad

3 (7-oz.) cans tuna fish
4 hard-boiled eggs, chopped
1 C. chopped ripe olives
1 small onion, minced
1 C. diced celery, diced

2 pkg. unflavored gelatin
½ C. cold water
2 C. mayonnaise
Parsley and celery curls,
   for garnish

Combine the tuna, eggs, olives, onion, and celery in a bowl and set aside. Soften the gelatin in the cold water and set over hot water and stir until dissolved. Stir in the mayonnaise. Add to tuna mixture and blend well. Turn into mold and chill until firm. Unmold and garnish with parsley and celery curls. Serves 10 to 12.

Crab-Stuffed Avocado

½ C. mayonnaise
½ C. celery, minced
¼ C. pimento, minced
2 tsp. lemon juice
⅛ tsp. Worcestershire sauce
Dash Tabasco (optional)

2 ripe avocados
2 tsp. lemon juice
⅛ tsp. salt
2 C. shredded crisp greens
1½ C. cooked or canned crab
   or lobster meat, chilled
Salad dressing of choice

In a bowl, combine the mayonnaise, celery, pimento, lemon juice, Worcestershire sauce, and Tabasco. Halve avocados lengthwise, remove pits, and peel. Sprinkle with lemon juice and salt. Arrange on a bed of crisp greens. Fill avocado halves with crab meat and top with a favorite salad dressing. Serves 4.

Salad Dressings

Salad dressings should all be homemade. While they enhance the salad, they can also contribute to good health. There is some doubt about using vinegar, though the number of readings prohibiting it is small. Lemon juice is preferred where acidity is desired. The oil used may be olive oil, frequently recommended in the readings, or vegetable oils. Olive oil is low in saturated fat, and in some quarters is considered a health food in its own right. Of the vegetable oils safflower oil is among the lowest in saturated fat and is high in vitamin E; sunflower oil, also low in saturated fat, is high in essential fatty acids; corn oil is reasonably low in saturated fat, with a high vitamin E content, essential fatty acids, and a small amount of B-complex vitamins. You might consider alternating oils or using a mixture of two or three vegetable oils to receive the benefits of each of them.

Avocados, used either in salad dressings or otherwise in the salad, are a nutritionally valuable addition. They are rich in protein, contain a highly digestible oil, and have vitamins A and C. Mineral content includes an ample amount of calcium, potassium, magnesium, and sodium, considerable iron and phosphorus, and smaller amounts of manganese and copper, essential to the assimilation of iron.

Avocado Dressing

1 avocado
Juice of 1 orange or 1 lemon

Whip the avocado pulp to the consistency of whipped cream. Add citrus juice very gradually, then whip with a rotary beater until light and frothy. Makes about 1 cup.

Mayonnaise

Mayonnaise is a great favorite, not only as a dressing but as an ingredient in other recipes. It is important to store all mayonnaise combinations in the refrigerator, as they are subject to bacterial growth that may be toxic without showing any evidence of spoilage. For those who prefer a mayonnaise without cholesterol, soy mayonnaise is available in natural food stores and some supermarkets. Plain yogurt also makes a good substitute in many recipes.

Mayonnaise #1

2 egg yolks	½ tsp. lemon juice
¼ to ½ tsp. dry mustard	½ C. salad oil: sunflower,
½ tsp. salt	safflower, peanut, etc.
Few grains of cayenne	3½ tbs. lemon juice

Be sure all ingredients are chilled. In a medium bowl, place the egg yolks, dry mustard, salt, cayenne, and ½ tsp. of lemon juice and beat with a wire whisk. Into the dressing, beat the salad oil very slowly, ½ tsp. at a time, alternately with the 3½ tbs. of lemon juice. Alternate adding the oil with a few drops of lemon juice, until all ingredients are incorporated. If the ingredients are cold and are added slowly during constant beating, this will make a thick dressing. Should the dressing separate, place one egg yolk in a bowl, stir constantly, and add the dressing very slowly. If the dressing is too heavy, thin it with a small amount of cream or whipped cream.

When making mayonnaise with an electric beater, beat the egg yolks at medium speed for 4 minutes. Combine the dry ingredients together and add them to the egg yolks. Add 1½ tbs. cold water. Add a half of the oil, drop by drop. When the dressing begins to thicken, add the lemon juice. Add the remaining oil more freely, beating constantly at medium speed. This should take about 20 minutes to make. Makes about 1 cup.

Mayonnaise #2

2 egg yolks
½ tsp. salt
2 tbs. lemon juice

¾ C. salad oil
2 tsp. honey (optional)

Put the egg yolks, salt, and lemon juice in a blender or food processor. Slowly add the oil while the machine is running, until desired consistency is reached. If using mayonnaise on fruit salads, add the honey. Makes about 1 cup.

Mayonnaise #3

2 egg yolks
2 tbs. lemon juice
½ tsp. salt
1 tsp. honey

½ tsp. dry mustard
Dash of cayenne
¾ C. salad oil

In a blender or food processor, combine the egg yolks, lemon juice, salt, honey, dry mustard, and cayenne. Add the salad oil very slowly, blending until thick. Makes about 1 cup.

French Dressing

1 C. salad oil
⅓ C. lemon juice
1 tsp. salt

¼ tsp. pepper
¼ tsp. garlic salt

In a blender or food processor, combine the oil, lemon juice, salt, pepper, and garlic salt and blend for 1 minute. Makes about 1⅓ cups.

Almond Nut Dressing

This is an excellent dressing for fruits, as well as vegetable salads.

2 tbs. almond butter   4 tbs. whole milk or cream

Beat the almond butter and milk together in a food processor or with an eggbeater until thoroughly blended. Makes about ⅓ cup.

Tomato Dressing

2 C. canned tomatoes   2 tbs. onion, grated
¾ C. lemon juice   1 tsp. vegetable broth powder
½ C. salad oil   1 tsp. paprika
¼ C. honey   2 cloves garlic, crushed
1 tbs. soy sauce

Sieve the tomatoes into a bowl and add the lemon juice, salad oil, honey, soy sauce, onion, vegetable broth powder, and paprika. Place in quart jar, shake well, and add the garlic. This will keep indefinitely in your refrigerator. Makes about 1 quart.

Peanut Butter Dressing

2 tbs. cold-pressed,   1 C. mayonnaise
   unhydrogenated peanut butter   1 tbs. salad oil
1½ tbs. lemon juice

In a food processor, combine the peanut butter, lemon juice, mayonnaise, and salad oil until well blended. Makes about 1¼ cups.

Yogurt or Sour Cream Dressing

1 C. sour cream or yogurt   ½ C. lemon juice

In a small bowl, combine the sour cream and lemon juice, and mix until well blended. This dressing is best with fruit salads but may be used on vegetable salads also. Makes about 1½ cups.

Yogurt and Honey Dressing

1 C. yogurt   Honey to taste

Combine yogurt and honey until well blended. Use as dressing on fruit salads. Makes about 1 cup.

3

Meats and Meat Substitutes

*I*ndividuals often asked Edgar Cayce whether or not to eat meat. The readings showed insight into the purposes and ideals of the questioners, while at the same time pointing out the need of the body for protein.

This, to be sure, is not an attempt to tell the body to go back to eating meat, but do supply, then, through the body forces, supplements, either in vitamins or in substitutes, for those who would hold to these influences—but purifying of mind is of the mind, not of the body. For, as the Master gave, it is not that which entereth in the body, but that which cometh out that causes sin. It is what one does with the purpose, for all things are pure in themselves, and are for the sustenance of man, body, mind, and soul, and remember—these must work together . . .   5401-1

(Q) Should the body abstain from meats for its best spiritual development?
(A) Meats of certain characters are necessary in the body-*building* forces in this system, and should not be wholly abstained from in the present. Spiritualize those influences, those activities, rather than abstaining. For, as He gave, that which

cometh out—rather than which goeth in—defileth the spiritual
body.   295-10

Scientific opinion favors eating meat for the purpose of body-
building, repair, and maintenance of repair functions; to obtain
vitamins, especially vitamin B; to acquire minerals, especially
phosphorus and iron; and to secure the important amino acids.
Meat, including poultry, fish, and eggs, has complete proteins. A complete protein is one that contains all the essential
amino acids (needed by the body to manufacture other proteins) in quantities readily usable by the body. One source of
complete protein from plants is the soybean; foods derived from
soy, such as tofu and tempeh, can be easily substituted for meat
in many recipes, for those who prefer not to eat meat.
The Cayce readings stress the use of meat in moderation, with
wild game preferable to domestic animals, and fish and fowl
preferable to red meat.

(Q) Please outline the proper diet, suggesting things to avoid.
(A) Avoid too much of the heavy meats not well cooked. Eat
plenty of vegetables of all characters. The meats taken would be
preferably fish, fowl and lamb; others *not* so often. Breakfast bacon, crisp, may be taken occasionally.   1710-4

In the diet keep away from red meats, ham, or rare steak or
roasts. Rather use fish, fowl and lamb . . .   3596-1

(Q) What should the diet be for this body?
(A) Not too much of meats of *any* character. Rather that . . . of
fowl or fish . . . those of the vegetable forces that give the clarify-
ing of blood forces; such as would be found in cooked onions,
beets, carrots or salsify, and in raw cabbage, of celery, of lettuce,
and these will act well with the mental and spiritual forces in
the body . . .   288-9

And in the matter of the diet, keep away from too much
greases or too much of any foods cooked in quantities of
grease—whether it be the fat of hog, sheep, beef or fowl! But
rather use the *lean* portions and those that will make for body-

building forces throughout. Fish and fowl are the preferable meats. No raw meat, and very little ever of hog meat. Only bacon. Do not use bacon or fats in cooking the vegetables . . .

                                                            303-11

Plenty of fowl—but prepared in such a way that more of the bone structure itself is as a part of the diet in its reaction through the system; that better reaction for the calcium . . . is obtained . . . Chew chicken necks, then. Chew the bones of the thigh. Have the marrow of beef, or such, as a part of the diet; as the vegetable soups that are rich in the beef carrying the marrow of the bone . . . and *eat the marrow!*   1523-8

In the diets: Keep away from heavy foods. Use those which are body building, as beef juice, beef broth, liver, fish, lamb, all may be taken but never fried foods.   5269-1

Surprisingly, we find high praise in the readings for wild game, which is seldom cited in nutrition tables. The readings caution about preparing rabbit or hare:

(Q) Is it all right for me to eat rabbit and squirrel, baked or stewed?

(A) Any wild game is preferable even to other meats, if these are prepared properly. Rabbit—be sure the tendon in both left legs is removed, or that as might cause a fever. It is what is called at times the wolve in the rabbit. While prepared in some ways this would be excellent for some disturbances in a body, it is never well for this to be eaten in a hare. Squirrel—of course, it is not in same. This stewed, or well cooked, is really more preferable for the body . . . but rabbit is well if that part indicated is removed.   2514-4

Eggs and cheese are also complete proteins. According to USDA bulletins, the important nutrients in eggs are protein, vitamin A (in the yolk), iron, vitamins B_1 and B_2. The readings also recommended eggs and cheese, with eggs frequently mentioned as a good breakfast food (see "Menus" chapter).

[Eggs] may be taken two to three times a week; any manner
save fried.   257-167

There are some elements in eggs not found in other foods,
ordinarily sulfur. The whites—however, do occasionally cause
certain other elements to be bad for the body. These we would
take occasionally, not necessarily avoiding same.
    (Q) Do I need any meat . . . ?
    (A) Not necessarily, if you are that minded. But remember, it is
what comes out—not what you take in—that defiles the body.
                                                          5399-1

Take as food values much that carries the iron, the silicon . . .
such as . . . beets, celery, radishes; all of those natures that give
the cleansing forces to the system. Spinach, eggs . . . Not too
heavy of meats, unless fish or fowl, or game. Never fried meats of
any character for *this* body . . . Broiled, boiled or baked, but not
with too much grease . . . Olives of every character . . . Cheese,
creams—all of this nature good for system.   257-11

The USDA Food Guide Pyramid recommends two to three
servings of dairy products per day, including milk, yogurt, and
cheese. It maintains that regardless of age, the calcium in milk
and other dairy products is important for good health.
    The readings recommended milk as a beverage for meals (see
"Menus" chapter) and gave milk as a source of calcium for those
who needed more in the diet. In addition, we have these side-
lights on the value of milk:

    . . . irradiated or dried milk . . . These as a whole are much
more healthful to most individuals than raw milk.   480-42

    Milk and all its products should be a portion of the body's
diet . . .   480-19

    . . . well that the general strength be builded up with beef
juices, egg and milk drinks, and the easily assimilated foods.
                                                          265-9

(Q) Is buttermilk good?

(A) This depends upon the manner in which it is made. This would tend to produce gas if it is the ordinary kind. But that *made* by the use of the Bulgarian tablets is good, in moderation; not too much. 404-6

Since milk and milk products and leafy green vegetables are rich in calcium and contain little starch, those who cannot tolerate milk but desire a nondairy source of calcium can eat dark leafy greens.

The Cayce readings give no explanation for the frequent recommendation of fish, fowl, and lamb, rather than red meats (with the exception of beef juice, which was often advised in cases of illness). It is recognized by nutritionists that fish, fowl, and lamb are more easily digested than beef and are a good source of complete proteins. Fish, especially ocean varieties, contain valuable minerals, particularly phosphorus and iodine, either not found in other meats or occurring in smaller quantities.

The readings also give no explanation for the statement that "Any wild game is preferable even to other meats . . . " (2514-4) Fish is a desirable food because commercial fertilizers and insecticides play no part in its production. Fish from the ocean are not injected with the hormones, antibiotics, or food adulterants prevalent in the meat industries. The same things could be said of game, which may be why it is highly recommended in the readings. Unlike in Cayce's time, today we must also keep in mind the effects of water pollution from chemical dumping, along with agricultural and industrial runoff.

The Cayce readings refer to glandular meats, such as tripe, calf's liver, brains, and the like, as "of the blood building [type] . . . " (275-24) The type of vitamins found more abundantly in the glandular meats are those that the bone marrow requires to produce red blood cells.

Cook all meats at low temperatures for maximum nutritive value, digestibility, and flavor. High temperatures toughen the protein and cause contraction of the fibers, squeezing out the meat juices. Fish and glandular meats in particular should be cooked at very low temperatures. These have very thin sheets of

connective tissue that break down around 150°; when they are
cooked above 150°, much of the juice is lost. Adding salt during
cooking also results in a loss of juice.

Meats should be roasted, baked, or broiled—never fried.
Stewing is permissible if the broth is to be used, in which case a
tightly covered pot should be used, with the meat being sim-
mered rather than boiled.

Broiling Temperature and Time

	Broiling temp.	Thickness or cut	Time (min.)
Fish steaks or fillets	Very low	1 to 1½ in.	15-18
Chicken, fryer or broiler	Low	Quarter or halved	45-50
Kidneys	Very low	½ in.	12-16
Lamb chops, patties,	Low	1 in.	20-30
or steaks	Low	2 in.	40-45
Milt	Low	Uncut	15-18
Rabbit, young fryer, 2 lb.	Low	Quartered	45-50
Liver	Low	¾ in.	12-18
Brains	Low	¾ in.	15-20

Baking or Roasting Temperature and Time

	Oven temp.	Internal temp. at which served	Time (min. per lb.)
Whole fish or fillets	300°	140°	1 in. thick 20 2 in. thick 30 3 in. thick 35
Chicken, roasting	300°	185°	35-40
Chicken, stewing	225°	185°	60-70
Duck, young	300°	185°	25-30
Goose, young	300°	185°	25-30
Lamb, leg	300°	155°-160°	25-30
Lamb, shoulder	275°	155°-160°	40-45
Rabbit	300°	180°	30-35
Turkey, large	300°	180°-185°	15-18
Turkey, small	300°	180°-185°	20-25
Liver, uncut	300°	145°-160°	15-20

Curried Cod Bake

2 lb. frozen cod, partly thawed
2 C. chopped onions
1 clove garlic, minced
2 tbs. butter or margarine
3 medium apples, pared, cored,

6 oz. tomato paste
¾ C. water
2 tsp. salt
1 tsp. curry powder
⅛ tsp. pepper
quartered, and sliced

Cut cod into 6 serving pieces, place in a 6-cup shallow baking dish. Sauté onions and garlic in butter or margarine in a medium skillet until soft; then stir in remaining ingredients. Heat, stirring constantly, to boiling; spoon over fish and cover. Bake in a 350° oven for 1 hour, or until fish flakes easily. Serves 6.

Poached Eggs and Broiled Fish

This is a high protein treat, since both fish and eggs are high sources of protein in addition to being fine sources of minerals and vitamins.

4 eggs
12 oz. broiled fish, cut into chunks

Paprika, for garnish

Poach the eggs in well-oiled muffin tins. Arrange the muffin-shaped eggs on a platter and surround them with chunks of broiled fish. Garnish with paprika. Serves 4.

Salmon Loaf

1 can salmon
1 tsp. lemon juice
1 can celery soup
3 tsp. chopped parsley

3 tsp. chopped green pepper
1 C. cooked peas
Dash of nutmeg

Combine all of the ingredients in a bowl, mixing to blend well. Transfer mixture to a lightly buttered loaf pan and bake in a pre-heated 350° oven for 30 minutes. Serves 4.

Quick-Baked Frozen Fish Fillets

This recipe is an exception to the rule that fish is better when fresh or thawed before cooking. It is included for those in a hurry.

1 lb. block frozen fish fillets
¼ C. unbleached flour
¾ tsp. salt
⅛ tsp. pepper

1 tsp. grated onion
3 tbs. melted butter
½ C. vegetable stock

Cut block of frozen fillets into quarters and set aside. In a shallow bowl, combine the flour, salt, and pepper. Roll the fish pieces in the flour mixture until well coated, then place in a well-greased ovenproof dish and set aside. Sauté the grated onion in the melted butter until softened, about 5 minutes. Stir in the vegetable stock. Pour the sauce over the fish, cover tightly, and bake in a preheated 325° oven for 20 to 25 minutes. Serves 4.

Red Snapper Fish Fillets

1¼ lb. red snapper fillets
2 cans tomato sauce, Spanish style
1 tbs. minced onion

1 tbs. minced parsley
Dash of cayenne

Place the fish fillets in an oiled baking dish. Pour tomato sauce over them. Sprinkle with onion, parsley, and cayenne. Place in preheated 300° oven for about 25 minutes or until fillets are cooked. Serves 5.

Fillet of Sole with Tomato-Herb Dressing

½ tbs. butter
3 tbs. finely minced onion
1 tbs. finely chopped green pepper
Juice of 1 lime
1 C. homemade mayonnaise

2 tbs. tomato paste
½ tsp. oregano
Pinch of savory
4 sole fillets
Lime juice, salt, and cracked
    pepper (for broiling fish)

Rub a warm skillet lightly with the butter. Add the onion and pepper and sauté over low heat until tender, about 8 minutes. Stir in the lime juice, mayonnaise, tomato paste, oregano, and savory and keep warm. Meanwhile, place the sole fillets on a broiler pan and sprinkle with additional lime juice, salt, and cracked pepper. Broil until just heated through, about 5 minutes. Serve topped with some of the sauce and place the remaining sauce in a bowl to serve on the side. Serves 4.

Baked Fish with Sour Cream

1 4-lb. whole whitefish   2 C. sour cream
1 tsp. paprika   Salt, to taste
1 tbs. butter

Split and remove bones from the whitefish. Flatten it out and rub inside and out with paprika and butter. Place fish in an ovenproof dish or shallow baking pan under the broiler and broil until it is lightly browned. Spread the sour cream over the fish, cover tightly, and bake covered in a 300° oven for 25 to 35 minutes. Remove from oven and season with salt. Serves 6.

Celery-Broiled Chicken

2 young broiling chickens   Cracked pepper, to taste
2 tbs. lemon juice   3 celery ribs, cut into strips

Split the chickens lengthwise and rub all over with lemon juice. Sprinkle with cracked pepper and place skin-side-down on a broiler pan. Place half of the celery strips in the cavities and broil for 10 to 12 minutes. Turn skin-side-up, place remaining celery strips over all and broil until browned and tender. Serves 4.

Broiled Chicken Fryers

1 fryer chicken, cut into pieces   ½ tsp. poultry seasoning
¾ tsp. salt

Combine the salt and poultry seasoning and rub the mixture

into the chicken pieces. Place the chicken pieces on the broiler rack and broil low in the oven until browned. Turn the chicken pieces and finish broiling until browned and until juices run clear when pierced with a fork. Serves 4.

Stewed Chicken

1 young chicken	1 tsp. salt
1 C. chopped celery tops	About 2 C. water

Select a young chicken that has a small amount of fat and place it in a pot with the celery, salt, and about 2 cups of water. Cover and cook over low heat, letting the water nearly cook away. Serve hot. Serves 4.

Chinese Turkey

2 tbs. butter or oil	1 C. chopped parsley
16 ribs celery, including leaves, chopped	24 julienne strips tangerine rind
1 C. chopped onion, lightly sautéed	1 15-lb. turkey
1 C. chopped mushrooms, lightly sautéed	¼ C. soy sauce
	1 C. honey
	¾ C. butter, unsalted

Heat the butter or oil in a large saucepan over medium heat. Add the celery and onion. Cover and cook until tender, about 5 minutes. Add the mushrooms and cook 3 minutes longer. Add the parsley and tangerine rind and stir to combine, then set aside. Wipe the interior of the turkey with soy sauce, stuff with the reserved dressing. Preheat oven to 450°. Make a paste of honey and butter and completely plaster the bird with this mixture, being careful to apply it under the wings. Place the turkey in a large pan and put it in the hot oven for 30 minutes or until it is evenly colored. Turn it several times with wooden spoons, being careful not to break the skin. Continue to brown until it is evenly crusted to a blackish brown. The honey turns black and, in carbonizing, completely seals the skin. Reduce the heat to 300° and roast for 3 to 4 hours. Baste with drippings after the first hour of cooking and every 20 minutes thereafter. Serves 10 to 12.

Roast Duck

1 3½- to 4-lb. domestic duck	½ tsp. salt
1 organic orange	1 tsp. honey
½ C. boiling consommé	1 tsp. lemon juice
1 C. boiling water	2 tbs. currant jelly,
3 tsp. brown sugar	plus more for garnish

Prepare the duck for cooking. Place it unstuffed on a rack in a pan. In a moderate oven (325°), roast the duck uncovered, allowing 20 to 30 minutes to the pound. Peel the orange and scrape the white pulp from the skin with a spoon and discard it. Cut the colored peel into very thin strips. Add a cupful of boiling water and simmer the peel for 15 minutes. Drain it, reserving the liquid. Remove all membrane from the orange sections and discard it. Fifteen minutes before the duck is done, pour the drippings from the pan and replace with the consommé. Continue to cook the duck and add to the drippings the orange liquid, salt, honey, and lemon juice. Simmer these ingredients for 10 minutes. Add the currant jelly and stir until dissolved. Add the orange peel and simmer 10 minutes longer. Add the consommé from the pan. Sprinkle the orange sections with the brown sugar and broil them for 3 minutes. Cut the duck into individual serving pieces and arrange on a hot platter. Garnish with orange sections and dabs of additional currant jelly and pour the sauce over it. Serves 4.

Roast Goose with Apple Dressing

1 C. currants or raisins
6 cooking apples
1 8-pound goose

Salt
2 tbs. water

Steam the currants or raisins in water in top of double boiler for 15 minutes. Peel, quarter, and core apples and combine them with currants or raisins and set aside. Prepare an 8-pound goose for cooking. (This weight is for a bird dressed but not drawn.) Rub the inside with salt and fill with the reserved dressing. If the bird is very fat, prick through the skin into the fat layer around the legs and wings. Truss the goose. Roast in a 325° oven on a rack in an uncovered pan, allowing 25 minutes per pound. Serves 8.

Chicken Cantonese

2 frying chickens, disjointed
¼ C. honey
¼ C. soy sauce

½ C. ketchup
¼ C. lemon juice

Arrange the chicken pieces in a single layer in a large baking dish. In a small bowl, combine the honey, soy sauce, ketchup, and lemon juice. Pour mixture over chicken pieces. Allow chicken to stand in marinade several hours or overnight. Cover pan and bake in a 325° oven for 1 hour. Remove cover and baste with sauce. Return to oven and bake uncovered until tender. Serves 6 to 8.

Roast Leg of Lamb

1 lamb leg
Powdered sea kelp

Mint leaves (optional)

Place the leg of lamb on a roaster rack with the fat side up. Rub it heavily with sea kelp. If you like mint with lamb, cut through the fat at intervals and pack mint leaves in the cuts. If you prefer other herbs, use them instead of the mint. Bake in a 300° oven, allowing 25 to 30 minutes per pound. Serves 8 to 10.

Broiled Lamb Chops and Potatoes

4 lamb chops

3 tbs. cooking oil

2 tsp. dried mint leaves or marjoram

1 tsp. powdered sea kelp

4 medium white potatoes

1 tbs. sesame seeds

Trim fat off the lamb chops or if, leaving any fat on, cut every ½ inch to prevent curling. Brush each chop with cooking oil and sprinkle with mint or marjoram and sea kelp. Place the chops in a shallow baking dish, cover, and allow to marinate in the refrigerator 4 to 6 hours. When ready to prepare dinner, place the chops on the broiler rack at room temperature while you prepare the potatoes. Scrub but do not peel the potatoes and cut into thin slices. Arrange potato slices on the broiler rack around the lamb chops. Brush with cooking oil and sprinkle with sea kelp. Broil the chops and potatoes slowly, turning the chops when browned on one side. Just before turning off the broiler, sprinkle the potato slices with sesame seeds and let them toast slightly. Serve chops and potatoes very hot. Serves 4.

Liver Dumplings and Dill Sauce

This is an excellent way to serve liver. The dumplings are very tender and can be eaten by small children and elderly people.

2 C. of liver

2 heaping tbs. cornmeal

2 eggs, beaten

1 tsp. fresh or dried marjoram

3 C. meat and vegetable stock

2 tbs. butter or cooking oil

1 tsp. dill seed

2 tbs. cold water

2 tsp. powdered sea kelp
1 tsp. minced onion

2 rounded tbs. of arrowroot
or cornstarch

Put the liver through a food grinder or food processor and place in a large bowl. Stir in the cornmeal, eggs, marjoram, sea kelp, and onion to make a stiff dumpling dough. Heat the stock in a large kettle and bring to a boil. When it boils, reduce heat to medium and dip a large tablespoon into the broth, then dip up a heaping spoonful of the dumpling batter, shaping it into a round ball with the spoon. Drop it into the boiling broth; dip the spoon into the broth again and repeat until you have 8 or 9 round liver dumplings distributed evenly in the boiling broth. Cover tightly and cook gently for 15 minutes without lifting the cover. Lift the dumplings out with a slotted spoon and place them in a serving bowl. Keep warm. Add the butter or oil and the dill seed into the broth. Combine arrowroot or cornstarch with cold water. Stir the arrowroot mixture into the broth, stirring until thickened. Pour this dill gravy over the liver dumplings and serve very hot. Serves 4.

Braised Liver

1 2-lb. piece liver
2 tsp. cooking oil
1 onion, sliced
2 tsp. Worcestershire sauce

2 tbs. ketchup
1 tbs. chopped green pepper
Salt and pepper, to taste
Hot water

Place liver in greased baking dish and brush sides with oil. Add onion, Worcestershire sauce, ketchup, green pepper, and salt and pepper to taste. Add enough hot water to nearly cover liver. Cover and cook at 300° for about 1½ hours. Remove lid for last 15 minutes of cooking time. Serves 6.

Molded Chicken Livers

1 lb. chicken livers
2 C. water
1 C. chopped celery leaves
1 tsp. powdered sea kelp

⅓ C. mayonnaise
1 hard-cooked egg, chopped,
    for garnish
½ medium onion, cut into
    rings, for garnish

Place the chicken livers in a saucepan with water, the celery leaves, and sea kelp. Bring to a boil and cook for 5 minutes or until livers are firm. Strain the broth and keep it for use as liquid for a molded or pressed meat dish later. Finely chop the livers and add mayonnaise. Place in a mold and chill. Serve with a sprinkling of chopped egg and onion rings. Serves 4 to 6.

Baked Brains

1 pair lamb or beef brains
1½ tbs. lemon juice
3 tbs. water
¼ C. whole wheat bread crumbs
2 hard-cooked eggs, chopped

1 tbs. ketchup
⅓ tsp. salt
⅛ tsp. pepper or paprika
4 tbs. cream
3 tbs. butter

Place the brains, 1 tbs. lemon juice, and the water in a sauce-pan and simmer for 15 minutes. Coarsely chop the prepared brains and place in a bowl. Add the bread crumbs, hard-cooked eggs, ketchup, remaining ½ tbs. lemon juice, salt, pepper, and cream and mix well. Transfer mixture to a greased baking dish or to individual dishes. Sprinkle the top with additional whole wheat bread crumbs. Dot with butter. Bake for 15 minutes at 400°. Serves 4 to 6.

Broiled Calf Brains on Tomatoes

1 pair calf brains	¼ tsp. salt
1 tbs. lemon juice	⅛ tsp. pepper
3 tbs. water	1 tsp. brown sugar
2 tbs. butter	2 tbs. whole wheat bread crumbs
8 thick slices of vine-ripened tomatoes	

Place the brains, lemon juice, and water in a saucepan and simmer for 15 minutes. Spread prepared brains with butter and place on a greased broiling pan rack. Broil the brains for 5 minutes on one side. Place tomato slices on an oven-proof plate, season tomato slices with salt, pepper, and brown sugar and cover one side with buttered whole wheat bread crumbs. Place the brains cooked-side-down on the tomatoes. Broil them for 5 minutes longer and serve at once. Serves 4.

Baked Rabbit

Although this recipe is for rabbit, pheasant or other wild game may be prepared in the same way.

1 rabbit	Juice of 1 lemon
½ tsp. salt	2 C. water
1 tbs. flour	½ lb. mushrooms
2 tbs. cooking oil	¼ C. butter
1½ C. sour cream	2 tbs. whole wheat flour

Cut rabbit into serving pieces (after tendons of left legs have been removed) and season with salt and flour. Brown quickly in oil. Arrange pieces in roaster pan. In a small bowl, combine ½ cup of the sour cream, the lemon juice, and ½ cup of water. Spread this sauce over the rabbit pieces. Bake uncovered at 300°, allowing 35 to 45 minutes per pound. While rabbit is cooking, sauté the mushrooms in the butter for about 15 minutes. Remove rabbit from pan and arrange on large platter. Add about 1

cup water to pan and heat, stirring to mix in all the meat juices.
In a bowl, combine the remaining 1 cup of sour cream, whole
wheat flour, and ½ cup of water. Add this to the meat juices to
make a light gravy. Add the cooked mushrooms to the gravy and
season to taste. Pour gravy over rabbit and serve. Serves 4.

Meat Substitutes

Complete proteins—those containing all the essential amino
acids—are necessary for building body tissue and thus maintaining good health. Also, many of the vitamins necessary to
health can be produced in the body itself only if a sufficient supply of these amino acids is present. It was commonly believed—
when the original recipe booklet was written—that to obtain a
sufficient amount of complete proteins was difficult without including meat or at least eggs and dairy products in the diet. Today, we know that in addition to animal sources, soybeans and
other soyfoods contain the essential amino acids and provide a
good source of protein without the cholesterol and saturated
fat of meat. We also know that far less of our diet needs to be
made up of protein than once was thought. This fact parallels
Cayce's dietary recommendations.

The following table gives the approximate amounts of complete proteins from animal and vegetable sources:

Animal	Amount	Gm. Protein
Milk, whole, skim, buttermilk	4 cups	32 to 35
Cottage cheese	½ cup	20
American or Swiss cheese	1 ounce	7
Meat, fish or fowl, boned	3 ounces	18 to 22
Egg	1	6

Vegetable	Amount	Gm. Protein
Soybean flour	1 cup	60
Cottonseed flour	1 cup	60
Wheat germ	1 cup	48
Brewer's yeast, powdered	¼ cup	25
Soybeans, cooked	½ cup	20
Tofu (soy product)	4 ounces	13

Vegetable	Amount	Gm. Protein
Tempeh (soy product)	4 ounces	20
Textured Soy Protein	½ cup	20
Nuts	½ cup	14 to 22

The protein of some nuts is incomplete. When combined with beans, grains, or dairy products, however, nuts can provide a more complete protein.

It is also possible to obtain complete proteins by combining foods that together provide essential amino acids. If the right combination of amino acids is consumed at the same meal, the body can build complete proteins. Combinations such as baked beans and brown bread or rice and beans supply many essential amino acids. To determine exactly which amino acids are contained in various foods would require considerable study. Therefore, it is important to include as many of the complete protein foods as possible in a meatless diet.

Carrot Loaf

1 C. mashed cooked carrots
1 small grated onion
2 tbs. oil or butter
½ C. peanut butter
2 C. cooked rice
2 eggs
1 can tomato paste

Salt and pepper, to taste
½ tsp. dried basil
2 tbs. butter
2 tbs. flour (or cornstarch)
1 C. cold water
2 tbs. chopped parsley,
 for garnish

In a bowl, combine the carrots, onion, oil or butter, peanut butter, rice, eggs, ½ can of the tomato paste, and salt and pepper to taste. Press mixture together as you would a meat loaf and place in a well-oiled baking pan and bake at 350° for 1 hour. Melt butter in a small saucepan over medium heat. Whisk in flour, stirring constantly. Combine the remaining ½ can of tomato paste with ½ cup of water and stir into flour mixture. Add salt and pepper to taste, along with the dried basil. Simmer sauce over low heat for 10 to 15 minutes and serve with the loaf, sprinkled with chopped parsley. Serves 4.

Carrot Burgers

Although this is a tasty way to eat carrots, if a burger is what you crave, there are many varieties of meatless burgers now available in supermarkets and health food stores that have the taste and texture of regular hamburgers.

1 C. grated raw carrots	2 raw egg yolks
1 C. ground walnuts	Raw peanut flour
1 C. ground sunflower seeds	2 tbs. cooking oil
1 tbs. chopped fresh herbs	

In a bowl, combine the carrot, walnuts, sunflower seeds, herbs, and egg yolks, mixing well. Shape mixture into 4 patties and roll in raw peanut flour. Heat oil in a skillet over medium heat. Add patties and cook until lightly browned on both sides. Serves 4.

Asparagus Soufflé

2 C. cooked asparagus, fresh or frozen	Salt, to taste
3 egg yolks	2 tbs. butter
1 C. cream	Water

Put cooked asparagus through a colander or purée in a food processor and blend with well-beaten egg yolks and cream. Add salt to taste and place in individual oiled molds. Place molds in pan to which ¼ inch of water has been added and bake in moderate 350° oven until custard is set, about 30 minutes. Add butter to each mold. Serve hot. Serves 4.

Sweet Potato Soufflé

2 C. mashed baked sweet potatoes
2 eggs, separated

1 tsp. salt
⅔ C. cream

Blend mashed sweet potatoes with beaten egg yolks, salt, and cream. Fold in stiffly beaten egg whites and transfer to a well-oiled soufflé dish. Bake in a 350° oven for 30 minutes. Serves 4.

Vegetable Loaf

2 lb. raw spinach
1½ C. grated carrots
1 onion, chopped
1 C. diced celery

1 green pepper, chopped
½ C. chopped nut meats
2 eggs, beaten
¼ C. vegetable oil

In a vegetable steamer, combine the spinach, carrots, onion, celery, and green pepper. Steam together until softened and transfer to a bowl. Add the chopped nut meats. In a small bowl, combine the beaten eggs and oil and add to mixture. Bake in a 350° oven for approximately 30 minutes. Serve with tomato juice. Serves 6 to 8.

Walnut-Lentil Loaf

1 C. lentils
1 C. chopped walnuts
½ C. chopped celery
1 small onion, minced

1 tsp. vegetized salt
1 egg, beaten
½ C. milk

Combine lentils, walnuts, celery, onion, and salt. Add the beaten egg and milk and mix until well combined. Transfer mixture to an oiled casserole and bake in a 350° oven for 1 hour. Serves 4.

Almond Nut Loaf

1 C. chopped celery tops   1 C. chopped apples
1 C. chopped celery   1 egg
1 C. chopped almonds   ½ C. milk

In a bowl combine the celery tops, celery, almonds, and apples. In a small bowl, beat the egg and add milk. Pour over mixture and blend well. Transfer mixture to an oiled loaf pan and bake in a 350° oven for 1 hour. Serves 4.

Nut Loaf Surprise

1 onion, chopped   1 tsp. soy sauce
1 C. chopped nut meats   Cottage cheese for desired
¼ tsp. paprika   consistency
1½ tsp. lemon juice

In a bowl, combine the onion, nut meats, paprika, soy sauce, cottage cheese, and lemon juice and mix well. Form into a loaf and pack firmly into a buttered loaf pan. Cover and chill in the refrigerator. Cut into slices and serve. Serves 4.

Nut Patties

¼ C. pecan butter (or other   2 tbs. minced parsley
   nut butter), thinned with water   1 tsp. vegetable broth powder
2 C. cooked grated carrots   ½ C. whole wheat toast crumbs

Thin nut butter with water to the consistency of a very thick sauce. Combine with the carrots, parsley, and vegetable broth powder, mixing well. Shape into patties. Roll in whole wheat toast crumbs, place on a buttered baking sheet, and bake in a 350° oven until brown. Serves 4.

Nut Loaf

1 C. finely chopped walnut meats	½ C. minced celery
1 C. dried whole wheat bread crumbs	1 garlic clove, minced
1 onion, finely chopped	1 egg, beaten
½ C. wheat germ	½ C. milk

In a bowl, combine the walnuts, bread crumbs, wheat germ, celery, garlic, and onion. In a small bowl combine the beaten egg and milk and pour this over the mixture, blending until well combined. Transfer mixture to an oiled loaf pan and bake 1½ hours in a 350° oven. Serves 4.

Large Nut Roast

½ C. minced onion	½ tsp. powdered sage
½ C. water	1 tbs. parsley, chopped
2 C. ground walnuts or pecans	Salt and garlic powder, to taste
1 C. whole wheat bread crumbs	2 eggs
1 C. wheat germ	1 C. milk
½ C. celery, chopped	Hot water and melted butter
4 tbs. butter	(for basting)

Pour ½ cup water in a skillet over medium heat. Add onions and cook for 5 minutes or until tender. Place onions in a bowl and add nuts, bread crumbs, wheat germ, celery, butter, sage, parsley, salt, and garlic. In a small bowl, beat eggs well, stir in milk, and pour over the mixture. Combine well and transfer mixture to an oiled baking dish. Bake at 350° for 30 to 45 minutes, basting with equal parts hot water and melted butter. Serves 6.

Spinach Nut Loaf

3 bunches cleaned spinach, chopped
1 C. chopped nut meats
2 eggs, well beaten
1 tsp. salt
1 small onion, chopped

½ C. finely chopped parsley
½ C. wheat germ
¾ C. whole wheat bread crumbs
2 tbs. butter
Tomato sauce (as topping)

In a bowl, combine the spinach, nut meats, eggs, salt, onion, parsley, wheat germ, and ¼ cup of the bread crumbs. Place mixture in an oiled loaf pan. Sprinkle remaining ½ cup bread crumbs over top, dot with butter, and bake in a 350° oven for about 30 minutes. Serve with your favorite tomato sauce. Serves 4.

Lima Bean Loaf

2 C. cooked lima beans
1 C. whole wheat bread crumbs
2 tbs. melted butter or oil
½ C. green peppers, chopped
½ C. onions, chopped

½ C. nuts, chopped
2 eggs, well beaten
½ C. milk or cream
Vegetable salt, to taste
Melted butter, for basting

In a bowl, combine the lima beans, bread crumbs, butter or oil, green peppers, onions, nuts, eggs, milk, and salt. Mix all ingredients together thoroughly and place in well-buttered loaf pan. Bake in a 350° oven for about 30 minutes or until done. Baste with melted butter. Serves 4 to 6.

Soybean Loaf #1

3 C. cooked soybeans, seasoned
½ tsp. dry mustard

2 tsp. raw sugar
½ C. hot water

2 tsp. sorghum, honey, or molasses

Mash cooked soybeans and place in a bowl. Add the mustard, sorghum, sugar, and water and mix well. Pour mixture into a well-oiled loaf pan and bake in a 350° oven until browned, about 30 minutes. Serves 4.

Soybean Noodles with Cheese

3 C. cooked soy noodles
½ C. diced canned tomatoes

2 tbs. vegetable broth powder
⅓ C. grated American cheese

Place noodles in an oiled baking dish and pour tomatoes over them. Sprinkle broth powder over noodles and then top with grated cheese. Bake in a 350° oven for 35 minutes. Serves 4.

Soybean Egg Loaf

½ lb. soybeans, cooked
2 eggs, beaten
2 tbs. chopped parsley

½ C. thinly sliced celery
1 small onion, chopped
1½ tsp. salt

Grind soybeans in a food processor. Add eggs, parsley, celery, onion, and salt and pulse to combine well. Transfer mixture to a well-oiled loaf pan and bake in a 350° oven for 30 minutes. Serves 4.

Soybean Loaf #2

3 C. cooked soybeans
1 small onion, chopped
1 tbs. salad oil
½ C. diced canned tomatoes

½ C. chopped green pepper
Salt and pepper, to taste
Tomato sauce (as topping)

Mash cooked soybeans and mix with onion, oil, tomatoes, green pepper, salt, and pepper. Transfer to an oiled loaf pan and bake for 1 hour at 350°. Serve with your favorite tomato sauce. Serves 4 to 6.

Eggs in a Nest

1 egg
⅓ C. milk
4 slices whole wheat bread,
   slightly dry

2 tbs. butter or margarine
1 10-oz. pkg. frozen spinach,
   cooked and drained
4 eggs, poached

Beat egg slightly with milk in a shallow bowl or pie plate. Dip bread slices in mixture turning to soak both sides well. In a large frying pan, sauté slowly in butter until golden, turning once. Top each slice with a ring of cooked, seasoned spinach. Place poached egg in center. Serve hot. Serves 4.

Cottage Cheese Patties

1 small onion, finely chopped
1 lb. cottage cheese

¾ C. whole wheat bread crumbs
⅓ C. wheat germ

In a bowl, combine the onion, cottage cheese, bread crumbs, and wheat germ until well mixed. Form mixture into small patties and bake on a greased baking sheet at 350° for 20 minutes. Serves 4 to 5.

Cheese Loaf

2 tbs. onion, chopped
2 tbs. butter
1 C. chopped walnuts or pecans

⅔ C. hot water
2 tbs. lemon juice
2 beaten eggs

½ C. whole wheat bread crumbs   Salt, to taste
½ C. wheat germ   Tomato sauce (optional)
1 C. grated cheese

Cook onions in ½ cup water for 5 minutes. Add butter, nuts, bread crumbs, wheat germ, cheese, hot water, lemon juice, eggs, and salt to taste. Mix well and transfer mixture to a well-oiled loaf pan and bake at 350° for 30 minutes. Serve with tomato sauce, if desired. Serves 4.

4

Whole Grain Breads and Cereals

*T*he readings advocated only whole grain cereals, used for breakfast or made into bread. There is also mention of buckwheat cakes and whole grain cereals prepared for breakfast, as well as whole wheat toast, and there are references to food values found in cereals and breads. The portions of two readings given below serve merely as an introduction to a whole body of information concerning whole grains.

> . . . rolled or crushed or cracked whole wheat, that is not cooked too long so as to destroy the whole vitamin force . . . this will add to the body the proper proportions of iron, silicon and the vitamins necessary to build up the blood supply that makes for resistance in the system. 840-1

> (Q) What is particularly wrong with my diet?
> (A) The tendencies for too much starches, pastries, white bread should be almost entirely eliminated. Not that you shouldn't eat ice cream, but don't eat cake too. White potatoes, such as macaroni or the like and cheeses, these eliminate. They are not very good for the body in any form. 416-18

It may be that case no. 416 was concerned about being overweight. Certainly the advice given him is good from a dietetic standpoint. Starches and sweets not burned up by activities are deposited as fat. Yet the focus of the Cayce reading is not upon obesity as such, but upon keeping the body healthy so that it can be a fit temple. The laws of balance and moderation hold true here as in all other aspects of living.

In the United States, wheat is the most popular grain for bread making, largely because its protein has the proper combination for forming gas bubbles, thereby making a light loaf. There are nutritional advantages as well, provided the grain is whole wheat, which means it contains both the bran and germ. Wheat, unlike other grains such as rye, will not grow in soil low in phosphorus; so all wheat has a fairly high content of this bone-building mineral, as well as silicon and iron. It is also an excellent source of the vitamin B complex, and wheat germ is the richest known source of vitamin E, important in maintaining a healthy cardiovascular system.

Many diet outlines in the readings included whole grain cereals and bread: "rolled or . . . cracked whole wheat," one recommended, "not cooked too long so as to destroy the whole vitamin force . . . this will add to the body the proper proportions of iron, silicon and the vitamins necessary to build up the blood supply that makes for resistance in the system." (840-1) Buckwheat cakes, rice cakes, and graham (whole wheat) cakes were also frequently recommended.

It is important that whole wheat flour be freshly ground, in order to protect the vitamin content. Deterioration of vitamins begins almost immediately after grinding, due to oxidation, and it is estimated that at least half the vitamin content may be lost within a few days' time, especially if the flour is not refrigerated. The oil of the wheat germ becomes rancid in a short time, impairing the flavor. Cracked wheat used for cereal is also best if cracked as shortly before use as possible. A small hand mill is useful for this purpose.

Wheat flour—being a starch—has an acid reaction that can be modified by adding carob, soy, or peanut flours to the wheat flour, as these three flours are alkaline producing.

Carob flour is produced from the pod of the carob tree, or honey locust, and is thought by some to have been the locust that John the Baptist ate in the wilderness; thus, it is called St. John's Bread. It has a sweet taste and pleasant flavor somewhat like chocolate and can be used as a substitute for both sugar and chocolate. It is low in starch, very high in natural sugars, and contains a large amount of minerals and a fair amount of several vitamins.

Soy flour is more than thirty-three percent protein, is extremely high in calcium (200 mg. per cup), has more iron, thiamin, riboflavin, and niacin than whole wheat flour, and is high in pantothenic acid, another important part of the vitamin B complex.

Peanut flour is even higher in protein, with one cup of flour (113 gm.) having 59 gm. of protein. It is also higher in calcium and thiamin than whole wheat flour and has twice the amount of iron and riboflavin and more than three times the amount of niacin than does whole wheat. Peanut flour has the added advantage that it can be used raw, and it has a flavor very pleasing to most people.

Breads

Yeast Breads

There are two important secrets to making good whole wheat bread. The first secret is to use fresh, stone-ground hard wheat flour, for it produces bread with superior flavor, texture, and nutritional value. If this kind of flour is not available, a family-sized stone grinding mill would be a worthwhile investment. Flour ground by roller mills contains larger particles of bran, which may irritate the digestive tract and make coarse bread; and the difference in flavor between freshly ground flour and that left standing in warehouses and on grocers' shelves is immense.

The second secret is to allow sufficient time after mixing and before baking for the bran particles to absorb moisture and become soft. This requires at least four hours, preferably longer, and is necessary to prevent the bread from being crumbly and dry.

Other factors influence the finished loaf of bread. The exact amount of flour needed to make dough of proper consistency for handling is best learned from experience. If measuring by volume, be aware that flour is packed more in some cases than others. Measurements in bread recipes are for unsifted flour; therefore, weighing the flour may give better results.

The exact temperature at which bread rises (80° to 85°) is important only if you wish rising time to be as short as possible. Otherwise, room temperature is usually satisfactory, and there is no danger of killing the yeast, which is possible when setting the dough in too warm a place, as in an oven.

Kneading time will vary with different flours. While the exact amount of kneading is important for the best possible texture in bread, it is not essential for good bread. In short, if good ingredients are used with reasonable care, it is difficult not to have bread superior in flavor and nutrition.

Whole Wheat Bread

5 C. lukewarm water	⅓ C. vegetable oil
1 pkg. or cake of yeast	½ C. honey
2 tbs. salt	3½ lb. (12 C.) unsifted whole wheat flour

Dissolve yeast in water, add salt, oil, and honey, and stir. Add flour all at once and stir until thoroughly mixed, then let stand for 20 minutes or longer before kneading. Knead on floured board until smooth and elastic and place in well-oiled bowl or pan (at least 6-quart size). Cover with plastic wrap and let rise to double its bulk. Punch down well to remove all gas bubbles. Continue to let rise, punching down each time as soon as double in bulk, until ready to make into loaves, preferably about 5 hours from time of mixing. It should rise at least twice in this time. Turn out on floured board, knead a few minutes, and divide into 4 equal portions. Knead and form into loaves, place in well-greased medium loaf pans, lightly grease top surface with vegetable oil, and cover loosely with plastic wrap. Let rise until not quite double in bulk and bake at 350° about 45 minutes. Makes 4 loaves.

Variations

#1. Dough may be mixed in the evening, using cold rather than lukewarm water and doubling the amount of yeast. Leave in the refrigerator overnight. In the morning, remove from refrigerator and let stand at room temperature 30 minutes, then knead and shape into loaves. Let rise and bake as in basic recipe.

#2. Mix in evening, omitting yeast, and let stand at room temperature overnight. In morning, soften two yeast cakes or two packages dry yeast in 2 to 4 tbs. warm water and add to dough mixture, working it in well with hands. Let dough rest 10 to 20 minutes, then knead, allowing to rise until double in bulk, and shape into loaves as above.

#3. If time does not allow for any of the above methods, yeast may be increased to 2 or 3 cakes, dough left in warm place to rise (be sure temperature is not above 85°) and kneaded and shaped into loaves after rising once to double in bulk, about 45 minutes or less. Bread will be less moist than in other methods.

#4. When bread has been formed into loaves, brush with water rather than oil, and sprinkle with sesame seed. This adds a delightful flavor and enhances the nutritional value.

#5. For increasing nutritional value, milk may be substituted for water (if fresh milk is used, it must be scalded), and soy flour substituted for part of the whole wheat flour (not more than ¼ the quantity, or 2 to 4 tbs.). Brewer's yeast may be added, but bread will probably not be as light, as the addition of substances not containing gluten decreases elasticity. Blackstrap molasses, which is extremely high in calcium, iron, and some of the B vitamins, may be substituted for all or part of the honey.

Whole Wheat Buns and Rolls

Buns and rolls may be made from the same dough as whole wheat bread. (Use ½ of the bread dough recipe to make 2 dozen rolls.)

Hamburger buns: Take pieces of dough the size of an egg. Roll each into ball and flatten to ¾ inch thickness. Place on oiled cookie sheet or shallow pan, allowing at least 1 inch between buns; brush with vegetable oil, cover with plastic wrap, and allow to rise until double or triple in size. Bake in a 350° oven for about 20 minutes. Makes 24 buns.

Rolls: Roll dough out on floured board to ½ inch thickness. Cut with biscuit cutter, dip in vegetable oil, and place close together in baking pan. Cover, let rise, and bake as above. Parker House rolls are shaped by holding left forefinger across center of round piece of dough, bringing far side of dough over, and pressing edges together. Makes 24 rolls.

Refrigerator Rolls

1½ C. lukewarm water	⅓ C. vegetable oil
2 pkg. or cakes yeast	2 eggs, well beaten
2 tsp. salt	4½ to 5 C. unsifted
⅓ C. honey	whole wheat flour

Dissolve yeast, salt, and honey in lukewarm water. Add oil and eggs and mix well, then stir in flour. Set in refrigerator overnight. Take dough from refrigerator about 2 hours before time for serving rolls, and let stand at room temperature about 30 minutes. Knead on floured board, shape, and let rise as above. Bake 15 to 20 minutes at 375°. Makes about 24 rolls.

Note: Scalded fresh milk or reconstituted powdered skim milk may be substituted for 1 cup of the water in this recipe, in which case the yeast and honey should be dissolved in the water (½ cup) and allowed to stand 20 minutes before adding other ingredients.

Wheat Germ Rolls

1 cake or pkg. yeast
1 C. warm water or milk
1½ tsp. salt
3 tbs. blackstrap molasses
1 egg

¼ C. vegetable oil
¾ C. toasted wheat germ
⅓ C. powdered milk
2½ C. whole wheat flour

Dissolve yeast in water or milk, add salt, molasses, egg, oil, wheat germ, powdered milk, and flour, and stir to mix. Then beat 200 strokes by hand or 10 minutes with an electric mixer. Cover bowl, and set in a warm place (not over 85°) until double in bulk. Make into rolls, kneading thoroughly and shaping as desired. When double or triple in bulk, bake at 350° for 20 to 25 minutes or until brown. Makes about 12 rolls.

Note: If time allows, this dough may be placed in refrigerator overnight as in recipe for Refrigerator Rolls (see recipe on p. 96), or, after rising, it may be stirred down and left in refrigerator for 1 to 8 hours before using.

Potato Rolls

2 pkg. or cakes yeast
1½ C. milk
½ C. potato water
4 tbs. honey
2 tsp. salt

2 eggs, beaten
⅓ C. mashed potatoes
4 tbs. vegetable oil
6 to 7 C. sifted
    whole wheat flour

Dissolve yeast in milk and potato water. Add honey, salt, eggs, mashed potatoes, and oil. Mix well and stir in 2½ cups flour to make a sponge. Let rise ½ hour. Add about 3½ cups flour to make a medium-stiff dough. Knead well and let rise until double in bulk. Knead again and shape into rolls. Put on well-greased pans, let rise 1 to 1½ hours, and bake for 20 minutes at 400°. Makes about 24 rolls.

Cinnamon Rolls

1 recipe roll dough	3 tbs. honey
1½ tbs. melted butter	2 tsp. cinnamon
1½ tbs. vegetable oil	½ C. raisins, pecans, or walnuts (optional)

Make dough as in either of foregoing recipes. Roll ¼ inch thick, brush with mixture of melted butter and vegetable oil, and dribble honey over surface. Sprinkle with cinnamon and with raisins, pecans, or walnuts, if desired. Roll like jelly roll, cut into 1-inch pieces, and set close together in baking pan. Let rise and bake at 350° for about 20 minutes. Makes about 16 rolls.

Coffee Cake

1 recipe roll dough	¾ tsp. cinnamon
¼ C. raw sugar or honey	¼ tsp. nutmeg
½ C. raisins	½ C. ground nuts
2 tbs. molasses or honey	

Combine ingredients of any of the roll dough recipes. Add the sugar and raisins and allow to rise according to roll dough recipe. After dough rises, roll it ⅓ inch thick, brush surface with molasses or honey, and sprinkle with cinnamon, nutmeg, and nuts, pressing nuts into dough. Let rise in refrigerator overnight. Bake in a 350° oven for 18 to 20 minutes. Serves 8 to 10.

Salad Sticks

Use any roll dough desired. Roll or pat dough to ½ inch thickness, cut into narrow strips, and brush with oil on all sides. Place 1 inch apart on greased baking sheet. Cover, let rise, and bake at 350° for 10 minutes. Makes about 24.

Raised Muffins

1 pkg. or cake of yeast	1 tsp. salt
1 C. warm water or milk	1 C. whole wheat pastry flour
3 tbs. honey or blackstrap molasses	½ C. wheat germ flour
3 tbs. vegetable oil	⅓ C. powdered milk

Dissolve yeast in water or milk and let stand for 5 minutes. Add honey, oil, and salt, and stir to combine. Sift in flour, wheat germ flour, and powdered milk. (Wheat germ may be substituted for wheat germ flour, but cannot be sifted.) Stir just enough to mix. Do not beat. Drop from tablespoon into oiled muffin pans until half full. Let rise until double in bulk. Bake at 350° for 20 minutes. Makes 12 large muffins.

Rye Bread #1

1 pkg. or cake of yeast	4 C. rye flour
2 C. warm potato water	2 C. whole wheat flour
1 tbs. salt	1 tsp. caraway seed
1 C. mashed potatoes	

Dissolve yeast in potato water, add the salt, potatoes, flours, and caraway seed. Stir to mix, and knead until smooth and elastic. Let rise in warm place until double in bulk. Form into loaves, place in pans, and let rise. Bake at 350° to 375° for 1 hour or until browned. Makes about 4 loaves.

Rye Bread #2

1 C. whole wheat flour	¼ C. honey
3 C. rye flour	1 cake yeast
1 tbs. salt	¼ C. lukewarm water
Hot water	

In a bowl, mix wheat flour, rye flour, and salt. While beating, pour in sufficient hot water to make a stiff batter. Cover and let stand until lukewarm. Add honey and yeast dissolved in the ¼ cup lukewarm water, and enough whole wheat flour to make a dough. Let stand until double in bulk, and shape into loaves. Let rise until double in bulk. Bake at 375° 1 hour or until loaves are browned. Makes about 3 loaves.

Rye Bread #3

¾ C. yellow cornmeal	1 pkg. or cake of yeast
1½ C. cold water	¼ C. lukewarm water
1½ C. boiling water	2 C. mashed potatoes
1½ tbs. salt	1 tbs. caraway seed
1 tbs. honey	2 C. whole wheat flour
2 tbs. vegetable oil	6 C. rye flour

Mix cornmeal with cold water in saucepan, add the boiling water, stirring constantly, and cook about 2 minutes to achieve a mushlike consistency. Stir in the salt, honey, and oil and let cool to lukewarm. Dissolve yeast in the lukewarm water and add to the cornmeal mixture, along with the potatoes, caraway seed, and flours. Mix well and knead on floured board to a smooth, stiff dough. Cover and let rise in a warm place until doubled in bulk. Divide into 4 parts, shape into loaves, and place in oiled pans. Let rise and bake 1 hour at 375°. Makes 4 loaves.

Pumpernickel

Follow directions of above recipe, substituting rye meal for the rye flour. Shape into small loaves and bake at 375° for 1 hour or until very well done. Makes 4 loaves.

Quick Breads

Quick breads are usually made light with baking powder. Since double-acting baking powder is made with an aluminum compound, it may not be wise to use it, even though it makes breads and cakes lighter. A non-aluminum brand, which is made with cream of tartar (a product of grapes) as its acid constituent, would be a better choice. Non-aluminum baking powders are available in natural food stores. A mixture of cream of tartar and soda (2½ tsp. of cream of tartar to 1 tsp. of soda for each quart of flour) may also be used for baking powder. Once the gas bubbles released by this combination escape from the dough or batter, no more are formed or released during cooking. So breads made with this type of baking powder must be handled quickly after liquid is added, and stirred as little as possible. For extra lightness, use more baking powder; an extra quantity of this type does not result in a bitter taste, as does baking powder made with aluminum.

It is the action of stirring or kneading wheat flour gluten that creates elasticity in bread. Stirring and kneading are desirable for yeast bread dough but not for quick bread dough, which will produce tougher bread if it is overhandled. Quick breads are more tender if made from soft wheat flour, which contains less gluten. Pastry flours are usually of this type. However, hard wheat flour, used for yeast bread, may still be used and can be more nutritious.

Buttermilk Biscuits

2 C. whole wheat flour	¼ tsp. soda
1 tsp. salt	⅓ C. vegetable oil
3 tsp. baking powder	¾ C. buttermilk

Sift the flour, salt, baking powder, and soda together in a bowl and mix in oil. Add the buttermilk all at once and stir quickly, only enough to mix. Pat dough out ½ inch thick on a floured board and cut with a biscuit cutter or floured glass. Brush biscuits with vegetable oil, place on a well-oiled baking sheet, and bake at 400° for 15 minutes or until lightly browned. Makes 12 biscuits.

Baking-Powder Biscuits

2 C. sifted whole wheat flour
1 tsp. salt
4 tsp. baking powder

6 tbs. vegetable oil
⅔ C. milk

Sift the flour, salt, and baking powder into a bowl and mix in oil thoroughly. Stir in milk to make a soft dough. Pat out on floured board, handling as little as possible. Cut with biscuit cutter or shape into squares with a knife. Place on a well-oiled baking sheet and bake at 375° to 400° for 15 minutes. Makes 12 biscuits.

Note: Butter can be substituted for part of the oil in either of these recipes for a richer flavor. For extra nutrients ½ cup wheat germ or wheat germ flour can be used in place of ½ cup flour. One-fourth cup powdered milk can be added, if desired.

Drop Biscuits

2 C. sifted whole wheat flour
1 tsp. salt
4 tsp. baking powder

6 tbs. vegetable oil
1¼ C. milk

Sift the flour, salt, and baking powder into a bowl and mix in oil thoroughly. Stir in milk to make a soft dough. Drop by spoonfuls onto oiled baking sheet or well-greased muffin tins. Bake at 375° to 400° for 15 minutes. Makes 12 biscuits.

Cheese Biscuits

2 C. sifted whole wheat flour
1 tsp. salt
4 tsp. baking powder

2 tbs. vegetable oil
⅔ C. milk
¾ C. shredded sharp Cheddar
cheese

Sift the flour, salt, and baking powder into a bowl and mix in oil thoroughly. Stir in milk to make a soft dough. Blend in shredded cheese. Pat out on floured board, handling as little as possible. Cut with biscuit cutter or shape into squares with a knife. Place on a well-oiled baking sheet and bake at 375° to 400° for 15 minutes. Makes 12 biscuits.

Wheat Germ Muffins

1 C. whole wheat flour
½ tsp. salt
3 tsp. baking powder
1½ C. wheat germ
1 C. milk

½ C. powdered milk
1 egg
¼ C. oil
¼ C. honey

In a bowl, sift together the whole wheat flour, salt, and baking powder, then add the wheat germ. In a separate bowl, mix together the milk, powdered milk, egg, oil, and honey. Combine the two mixtures. Stir quickly and spoon into buttered muffin tins. Bake for 20 minutes at 400°. Makes 1 dozen large muffins.
Note: Raisins, chopped dates, or nuts may be added, if desired.

Dried-Fruit Muffins

2 eggs, separated
2 tbs. oil

1 C. chopped figs, prunes,
and raisins

1 tbs. maple syrup   ½ C. wheat germ
1 tsp. sea kelp   ½ C. peanut flour

Beat the egg whites stiff and set aside. Blend the egg yolks, oil, maple syrup, sea kelp, chopped dry fruit, wheat germ, and peanut flour, and fold in the egg whites last. Pour batter into oiled muffin tins and bake about 25 minutes at 350°. Makes 6 large muffins.

Note: The cup of dried fruit may be of any variety, just so there is a cup of packed dried fruit after chopping. This recipe may be easily doubled if desired. These are fine breakfast muffins.

Corn-Caraway Gems

2 eggs, separated   2 tbs. cooking oil
1 tbs. honey   ½ C. wheat germ
1 tsp. caraway seed   ½ C. coconut or nut milk
1 tsp. powdered sea kelp   ¾ C. yellow corn flour

In a bowl, combine the egg yolks, honey, caraway seed, sea kelp, oil, wheat germ, nut milk, and corn flour. Beat the egg whites stiff and fold into the mixture. Bake in tiny muffin tins, if possible, or in small custard cups. Have baking dishes well oiled and bake about 10 minutes at 400° or until brown and done in the middle. These are crunchy and very good. Makes 6 to 12 muffins (depending on size of tins).

Hot Cakes

1½ C. unsifted whole wheat flour   1 egg, beaten
3 tsp. baking powder   2 tbs. honey or raw sugar
½ tsp. salt   3 or 4 tbs. oil
1¼ C. milk

Sift the flour, baking powder, and salt together in a bowl and set aside. In a blender, place the milk, egg, honey, and oil and blend well. Combine the two mixtures, stirring just enough to mix. Cook on slightly oiled hot griddle. Serves 2 or 3.

Buckwheat Cakes

1 C. milk
1 C. cooked brown rice
2 eggs, separated
¾ C. buckwheat flour

1 tsp. baking powder
½ tsp. salt
1 tbs. melted butter
Butter and maple syrup (as toppings)

Blend milk with rice, and add well-beaten egg yolks. Combine the flour, baking powder, and salt into this mixture and add the butter. Whip egg whites until stiff and fold into the mixture. Cook on oiled griddle and serve with butter and maple syrup. Serves 4.

Wheat Germ Pancakes

For directions on making nut milk, refer to chapter six on beverages. Almond milk is also available at natural food stores in convenient 1-quart aseptic containers.

4 eggs, separated
2 C. nut milk
1 C. brown rice flour
2 tbs. cooking oil

1½ tsp. powdered sea kelp
1 tsp. honey (optional)
2 C. wheat germ

Beat the egg yolks, then add the milk and flour. Beat well, adding the oil, sea kelp, honey, and wheat germ. Fold in the stiffly beaten whites of the 4 eggs just before cooking on an oiled griddle. Makes 16 nutritious pancakes.

Waffles

1 C. sifted whole wheat flour
3 tsp. baking powder
½ tsp. salt
2 eggs, separated

1¼ C. milk
¼ C. oil
2 tsp. raw sugar or other
   natural sweetener

Sift flour, baking powder, and salt 3 times. Beat together the egg yolks, milk, oil, and sugar, and continue beating 2 minutes with an electric mixer on low speed. Fold in beaten egg whites and bake in preheated waffle iron. Serves 2.

Buckwheat Waffles

2 C. water
1 tsp. lemon juice
¼ C. soy flour or powder
1¼ C. buckwheat flour
2 tbs. honey
¼ C. raw almonds

3 tbs. vegetable oil
¾ tsp. sea salt
¼ C. oatmeal
¾ C. whole wheat flour
2 tbs. molasses

In a blender, combine water with the lemon juice. Add soy flour, buckwheat flour, honey, almonds, oil, salt, oatmeal, whole wheat flour, and molasses. Mix thoroughly and bake in a preheated waffle iron. Serves 4.

Nut Waffles

1 C. whole wheat flour
¼ C. soy flour
¾ tsp. salt
3 tsp. baking powder
1¼ C. sweet milk

2 eggs, separated
2 tbs. raw sugar or honey
5 tbs. oil
¼ to ½ C. chopped pecans
   or almond milk or other nuts

Sift wheat flour, soy flour, salt, and baking powder twice. In a separate bowl, combine the milk, egg yolks, sugar, and oil. Combine the two mixtures, add the chopped nuts, and fold in the egg whites. Mix thoroughly and bake in a preheated waffle iron. Serves 4.

Spicy Apple Bread

1 C. unsifted whole wheat flour
1 tsp. soda
1 tsp. salt
1 tsp. cinnamon
½ tsp. nutmeg
½ tsp. cloves
½ C. butter

¾ C. dark brown sugar
2 eggs, beaten
1 C. coarsely grated sour apples
1 C. unsifted whole wheat flour
¼ C. sour milk or buttermilk
½ C. chopped nuts

Sift together first six ingredients and set aside. In mixing bowl combine the butter, sugar, and eggs and beat well. Stir in the apples and the second cup of flour. Add the sour milk and blend well; add the sifted ingredients and stir just until well mixed. Add the nuts and bake in a greased 9"x5"x3" loaf pan at 350° for 55 to 60 minutes. Allow to cool for several hours before slicing. Makes 1 loaf.

Date-Nut Bread

2 C. boiling water
1 tsp. soda
2 C. chopped dates
2 tsp. butter
2 eggs, beaten
2 C. raw sugar or other
   natural sweetener
4 C. sifted whole wheat flour

½ tsp. salt
2 tsp. cinnamon
3 tsp. baking powder
1 C. chopped nuts
   (preferably pecans)
2 tsp. vanilla
1 C. raisins (optional)

Combine boiling water and soda, then add dates and butter. Combine beaten eggs and sugar and add to first mixture. Add flour, salt, cinnamon, and baking powder, which have been sifted together twice. Add nuts and vanilla. Raisins may be added if desired. Pour into loaf pans and let stand for 5 minutes. Bake 1 hour and 15 minutes at 325° to 350°. Loaf pans should be greased and the bottom lined with waxed paper. Makes 2 loaves.

Nut Bread

1 C. warm potato water	1 C. raisins
1 pkg. dry yeast	1 egg, beaten
1 C. corn flour	1 tbs. oil
2 tsp. honey	1 C. peanut flour
½ C. sunflower seed meal	1 C. wheat germ flour
1 C. chopped nuts	1 tsp. powdered sea kelp

In a bowl, combine the potato water, yeast, corn flour, and honey. Blend mixture together and let rise until very light, about 45 minutes. Then add the sunflower seed meal, chopped nuts, raisins, egg, oil, peanut flour, wheat germ flour, and sea kelp to make a stiff loaf. Do not knead this bread, because it contains no gluten. Stir with a big spoon, then put into an oiled loaf pan. Let rise while the oven heats and bake 10 minutes at 400°, then about 50 minutes at 350°. Makes 1 loaf.

Steamed Date-Nut Bread

This bread is extremely high in protein, calcium, iron, and the B vitamins.

1 C. whole wheat flour	½ C. pecans
1 C. soy flour	2 C. buttermilk
3 tsp. bone meal	¾ C. blackstrap molasses
1½ tsp. soda	1 tbs. vegetable oil

1 C. wheat germ   3 tbs. Tortula yeast
1 C. dates

Sift together the wheat flour, soy flour, bone meal, and soda. Add the wheat germ, dates, and pecans. In a separate bowl, combine the buttermilk, molasses, oil, and yeast, and combine both mixtures together quickly, stirring as little as possible. Pour into greased molds, filling about ⅔ full, cover, and steam for 2 hours. Five 20-ounce (2½ cup) cans may be used as molds. Makes 5 loaves.

Steamed Brown Bread

1 C. All-Bran cereal   ½ C. sugar
1 C. sour milk   1 C. whole wheat flour
½ C. raisins   1 tsp. soda
1 tbs. molasses   ¼ tsp. salt

Mix All-Bran, sour milk, and raisins. Let the milk get absorbed, then add the molasses, sugar, flour, soda, and salt. Put into a tall greased coffee can. Cover tightly and steam 3 hours. Makes 1 loaf.

Dixie Corn Bread

4 C. soy milk   2 tbs. cooking oil
2 C. yellow cornmeal   1 tsp. powdered sea kelp
4 eggs, separated

Heat the milk until hot and add the cornmeal gradually, stirring constantly. Stir and cook until very thick. Remove from heat and cool until just warm. Beat the 4 egg whites stiff, then beat the cornmeal mixture with the egg yolks, oil, and sea kelp, blending thoroughly. Fold in the egg whites and pour the batter into an oiled rectangular cake pan. Bake at 375° until done, about 45 minutes. Makes 1 pan.

Whole Wheat Cornmeal Bread

1 C. cornmeal	⅓ C. shortening
1 C. whole wheat flour	1 C. milk
2 tsp. baking powder	1 egg
1 tsp. salt	¼ C. sugar

In a bowl, combine the cornmeal, flour, baking powder, and salt. In a separate bowl, combine the shortening, milk, egg, and sugar. Combine both mixtures and blend well. Pour the batter into an oiled rectangular cake pan. Bake at 375° until done, about 45 minutes. Makes 1 pan.

Peanut Bread

These raw slices of nut bread are delightful in flavor and high in nutrition. Made very tiny, they may be served as hors d'oeuvres, as between-meal snacks, or as children's afternoon treats.

2 C. raw peanut flour	1 C. ground nuts (preferably
¼ C. homemade (or	black walnuts)
unhydrogenated) peanut butter	3 tbs. soy or nut milk

In a bowl, combine the peanut flour, peanut butter, ground nuts, and soy or nut milk. Add extra peanut butter if mixture is too dry, or peanut flour if it is too sticky. Shape into thin wafers and arrange on a cookie sheet. Allow to dry at room temperature for 30 minutes, then store in a covered container. Makes about 48 wafers.

Oatmeal Crackers

1 C. cold potato water   4 C. quick-cooking oatmeal
½ C. cooking oil   ½ C. sesame seeds
1 tsp. powdered sea kelp

In a bowl, combine the potato water, oil, sea kelp, and oatmeal, mixing well to form a stiff dough. Place in the refrigerator to chill. Lightly flour a board and roll the dough thin. Sprinkle with sesame seeds and press these into dough with rolling pin. Cut dough into squares and bake on oiled cookie sheet at 350° for 25 minutes. Makes about 48 crackers.

Whole Wheat Crackers

3 C. sifted whole wheat pastry flour   ½ C. vegetable oil
1 tsp. (scant) sea salt   ⅓ C. plus 3 tbs. soy milk

Sift flour and salt together, add oil and mix well. Add soy milk, and mix to stiff dough. Roll thin, cut in desired shapes, and prick with a fork. Bake at 350° until brown, at least 20 minutes. Makes about 48 crackers.

Health Crackers

2 C. whole wheat pastry flour   ¾ tsp. sea salt
1 C. millet meal   ¾ C. vegetable oil
½ C. rice polishings   2 tbs. honey
¼ C. sunflower seed meal   ¾ C. water

Combine the flour, millet meal, rice polishings, sunflower seed meal, and sea salt in a bowl, mixing well. Add the oil and blend in well using fingers or pastry cutter. Mix in honey dissolved in the water and knead slightly. Roll to the thickness of a piecrust. Cut into squares and prick with fork. Bake at 350° until brown, about 20 minutes. Makes about 48 crackers.

Cereals

Whole Wheat

2 C. water   1 C. whole wheat
1 tsp. salt

Bring water to a boil and add salt and wheat. Remove from direct heat as soon as water reaches second boil, pour into casserole dish and place uncovered on adapter ring or shelf of steamer. Have boiling water in bottom of steamer to within 1 inch of the steamer shelf. Cover steamer tightly and cook over low heat to keep water in steamer just simmering for about 8 hours, checking water level occasionally and adding more water when necessary. Serve with butter or cream and honey. Serves 2 or 3.

Cracked Wheat

1 C. cracked wheat   1 tsp. salt
4 C. water

Add salt and cracked wheat to boiling water and cook over direct heat for about 30 minutes or in a double boiler for 1 hour or more. This may be started in double boiler at night and cooked for 30 minutes, then finished cooking in the morning.

An alternative cooking method, which would retain more vitamins but possibly make the wheat less digestible, is as follows:

Add 1 cup cracked wheat to 3 cups boiling salted water. Boil for 5 minutes, then put into a 1-quart thermos to retain heat, and leave for 8 hours before serving.

Multigrain Dry Cereal #1

3 C. whole wheat flour	1½ C. dry malt
3 C. cornmeal	3½ C. milk or soy milk
3 C. millet flour	4 tbs. honey
3 C. oatmeal	1 tbs. salt or sea salt

In a large bowl, combine the wheat flour, cornmeal, millet flour, oatmeal, and salt. Mix well. In a separate bowl, combine the milk, malt, and honey, and add to dry ingredients to make a stiff dough. Roll out very thin, prick, and bake on a sheet pan at 300° until golden brown. Pulse in a food processor to crumble it. Makes about 12 cups.

Multigrain Dry Cereal #2

1 C. whole wheat flour	1 tbs. sea salt
½ C. rye flour	½ C. water
1 C. soy flour	½ C. honey
½ C. cornmeal	½ C. oil
1 C. oatmeal	3 tsp. toasted sesame seeds
½ C. rice bran	

In a bowl, combine the wheat flour, rye flour, soy flour, cornmeal, oatmeal, rice bran, sea salt, and sesame seeds. In a separate bowl, combine the water, honey, and oil, and add to the dry mixture, stirring to form granules. Bake on a sheet pan at 325° until lightly browned, stirring frequently. Turn off oven and allow cereal to stay in oven, stirring occasionally until cool. Makes about 6 cups.

5

Desserts and Sweets

Some of us have more of a "sweet tooth" than others. The readings recognized this desire for sweets and gave the following advice:

(Q) Suggest best sugars for body.
(A) Beet sugars are the better for *all,* or the cane sugars that are not clarified.   1131-2

Keep away from too much sweets though honey may be taken.
                                                                        3053-4

Keep the body from too much sweets—though *sufficient . . .* to form sufficient alcohol for the system; that is, the kind of sweets, rather than sweets. Grape sugars—hence grape jellies, or of that nature are well.   487-11

Do be careful that there are not quantities of pastries, pies, or candies, especially chocolate nor carbonated waters. These, as we find, will be hard on the body . . .   5218-1

Saccharin may be used. Brown sugar is not harmful. The *bet-*

ter would be to use beet sugar for sweetening.   307-6

(Q) What type of sweets may be eaten by the body?
(A) Honey, especially in the honeycomb; or preserves made with *beet* sugar rather than cane sugar. Not too great a quantity of any of these . . . but the forces in sweets to make for the proper activity through the action of the gastric flows . . . for these become body-building in making for the proper fermentation (if it may be called so) in the digestive activities. Hence two or three times a week the honey upon the bread . . . would furnish that necessary in the whole system.   808-3

Energies or activities may burn acids but those who lead the sedentary life or the non-active life can't go on sweets or too much starches—but these should be well-balanced.   798-1

The diet also should be considered—in that there is not an excess of acids or sweets, or even an excess of alkalinity . . .
There should be kept a normal, well balanced diet that has proven to be right for the individual body.   902-1

The kind of sweet taken is important, as well as the amount. Those sweets recommended were grape sugars, beet sugars, raw cane sugars, and honey, especially in the honeycomb. Another natural sweetener—date sugar—is now available.

With regard to chocolate, one reading recommended "Chocolates that are *plain*—not those of any that carry corn starches should be taken, or [not] those that carry too much of the cane sugar." (487-11) Several later readings, however, warned against chocolates made during the war years. Said one, given in 1944, "Chocolate that is prepared in the present is not best for *any* diet." (4047-1)

While scientific sources have not confirmed the statement in the Cayce readings that beet sugar is preferable to cane sugar (or that there is any difference, from a chemical standpoint), the deleterious effects of refined sugars and concentrated sweets in excessive amounts are widely recognized.

According to Adelle Davis, one of the country's best-known nutritionists, excessive eating of sweets, especially refined sugar, increases the need for choline. A deficiency of choline has been found to produce nephritis and liver damage; it also interferes with the absorption of calcium by increasing the production of alkaline digestive juices. This alkalinity counteracts the acidity of the digestive juices of the stomach necessary to dissolve calcium. Davis also notes that people suffering from atherosclerosis often report a particularly high intake of refined sugar.

J. I. Rodale, former editor of *Prevention* magazine, asserts that consuming refined sugars makes one susceptible to insect bites, sinus trouble, stomach trouble, arthritis, pyorrhea, dental decay, and cancer. Eating refined sugar depletes B vitamins. While B vitamins occur in the natural sweets, fruits, and sugar cane and are necessary for the assimilation of sugars, when refined sugars are eaten, these vitamins are drawn from the organs and tissues of the body, leaving them deficient in these important food substances.

According to *The Nutrition Desk Reference* by Robert Garrison, Jr., M.A., R.Ph., and Elizabeth Somer, M.A., R.D. (Keats Publishing, 1995), the average American eats over 130 pounds of sugar per year, which amounts to forty teaspoons per day. Sugar contributes indirectly to malnutrition, as it supplies calories without nutritional benefits. Sugar has been linked to a variety of diseases, including obesity, cardiovascular disease, cancer, and diabetes. In addition, sugar is probably most infamous for its association with tooth decay in all ages, gum disease, and eventual loss of teeth.

Melvin Page, D.D.S., in his book *Degeneration-Regeneration*, states that sugar is indirectly a cause of dental decay, pyorrhea, and arthritis, in that it disturbs the calcium-phosphorus balance. Sugar disturbs this balance, he says, more than any other single factor. The amounts of these materials, he believes, is not as important as their proportions to each other. He also states that he does not recall a single cancer case that showed correct sugar level of the blood.

In her book *Lick the Sugar Habit* (Avery, 1996), Nancy Appleton, Ph.D., asserts that sugar can actually suppress the immune system and upset the body's mineral balance. Sugar is said to cause a copper deficiency, may lead to a chromium deficiency, and interferes with absorption of calcium and magnesium. Dr. Appleton further states that sugar can raise adrenaline levels in children and cause arthritis, asthma, candidiasis, varicose veins, and appendicitis. Other sugar-spawned maladies include a decrease in insulin sensitivity, a decreased glucose tolerance, an increased cholesterol level, nearsightedness, and hypoglycemia (low blood sugar).

Hypoglycemia is related to a wide variety of ills, including asthma, alcoholism, neuroses, fatigue, rheumatic fever, ulcers, epilepsy, and depression.

All sweets, save natural sweets such as those found in most fruits, maple syrups, and honey, are acid producing, another reason to limit the consumption of them. Fruits (fresh, stewed, or dried), confections, and desserts made with dried fruits and honey as the only sweetening agent, and honey used on bread and cereals can supply the sugars necessary to form the alcohol needed for proper digestion and assimilation; they are also the sources of sugar recommended from a nutritional standpoint, although an excess of these can also produce an unhealthy imbalance.

Raw sugar was among those sweets recommended in the Cayce readings. Real sugar (that is, sugar which has not gone through the refining process) is now impractical to obtain in this country. That which is sold as raw sugar at the present time is called Turbinado sugar and is produced by adding molasses to refined white sugar, thereby replacing the vitamins and minerals removed in the refining process.

There is also a host of sweeteners available in natural food stores, including honey, molasses, brown rice syrup, and barley malt. Another high quality sweetener is Sucanat, made by extracting the juice from sugar cane, which is then milled into a powder. This process retains the vitamins and minerals.

Since most people enjoy eating some cookies, cakes, and other desserts, this book includes dessert recipes that use raw sugar and other natural sweeteners. However, it would be wise to remember the caution in the readings against the combination of starches and sweets.

Protein Cake

7 eggs, separated   ½ lb. nut meats, ground fine
1 C. raw or brown sugar or   Pinch of salt
   ½ C. of each   1 tsp. vanilla

Beat egg whites until very stiff and dry. Set aside. Beat egg yolks and sugar together until creamy, add nut meats gradually, then add salt and vanilla. Fold this mixture into the egg whites carefully, and bake in an ungreased tube pan for 1 hour at 325°. Invert pan to cool. Makes 1 cake.

Caramel Sauce

⅔ C. maple syrup   4 tbs. cream
⅔ C. brown sugar   1 tbs. butter

In a saucepan, combine the maple syrup, brown sugar, and cream. Simmer for 2 to 3 minutes, allow to partially cool, then stir in the butter, and finish cooling. Makes about 1½ cups.

Carob Cake

½ C. butter   ½ tsp. cinnamon
1 C. raw sugar or   ½ tsp. baking powder
   other natural sweetener   ½ tsp. baking soda
2 eggs   ½ tsp. salt
1 C. sifted whole wheat pastry flour ½ C. buttermilk
½ C. carob powder   1 tsp. vanilla

Cream the butter and sugar, add eggs, and beat well. In a separate bowl, combine the flour, carob powder, cinnamon, baking powder, baking soda, and salt. Sift dry ingredients together three times. Add sifted dry ingredients to the creamed mixture, alternating with buttermilk and vanilla, beating well. Pour into an oiled 8"x8" baking pan and bake at 350° for 25 to 30 minutes. Frost with Carob Fudge Frosting (see recipe below). Makes 1 cake.

Carob Fudge Frosting

¾ C. rich milk   ¼ C. butter
¼ C. carob powder   2 C. raw sugar or
                                      other natural sweetener

Place the milk, carob powder, and butter in a saucepan over medium heat, stirring constantly until smooth and thick. Add the sugar and stir until completely dissolved. Without stirring, cook until the "soft ball" stage when tested in cold water. Frost cooled cake. Makes about 2 cups.

Oatmeal Cake

1 C. oatmeal   1 tsp. vanilla
½ C. boiling water   ½ tsp. salt
½ C. chopped dates or raisins   1 tsp. baking soda
½ C. butter   1½ C. whole wheat flour
2 eggs

Pour boiling water over the oatmeal and dates or raisins. Stir well and cool. After it is cooled, stir and add the butter, eggs, vanilla, salt, baking soda, and flour to the oatmeal and fruit mixture, mixing well. Transfer batter to a well-oiled cake pan and bake at 375° for 30 minutes. Makes 1 cake.

Topping

¼ C. butter

2 tbs. water

¼ C. whole wheat flour

¾ C. nuts or coconut

½ C. brown sugar

In a saúcepan, melt the butter and add the water, flour, sugar, and nuts or coconut, mixing well. Spread topping over the cake and return to oven for about 10 minutes. Makes about 1½ cups.

Deluxe Spice Cupcakes

1 C. boiling water

1 C. uncooked prunes or
   dates, pitted and chopped
   (or 2 cans applesauce)

2 C. unsifted whole wheat flour

1½ C. dark brown sugar

1 tsp. salt

1¼ tsp. soda

1 tsp. each: cinnamon,
   nutmeg, cloves, ginger, allspice

3 eggs

1 C. raisins (optional)

½ C. vegetable oil

Pour boiling water over the prunes or dates. Let stand a minimum of 2 hours. (Omit this step if using applesauce.) Place fruit mixture and all other ingredients (except raisins) in small bowl of mixer. Blend for 1 minute at low speed. Beat 2 minutes at medium speed. Add raisins and stir in. Place cupcake liners in 24 cupcake tins and divide batter among them. Bake 25 minutes at 350°. When cool, sift over top of cakes: 1 part dried milk to 1 part powdered sugar. Makes 2 dozen cupcakes.

Peanut Cookies

These cookies make a high protein dessert or snack to satisfy the peanut lover's taste for peanuts. Easily digested, both children and the elderly can enjoy them.

1 C. chopped,
    organically grown peanuts
½ C. homemade (or
    unhydrogenated) peanut butter
1½ C. peanut flour

Sunflower seed meal
    (for rolling)
Salad oil or soy
    milk powder (optional)

In a bowl, combine the peanuts, peanut butter, and peanut flour, mixing well. If too dry, add a few drops of salad oil. If too sticky, add a bit of soy milk powder. Shape into small cookies and roll in sunflower seed meal. Store in the refrigerator. Makes about 24 cookies.

Nutty Confections

¼ lb. of brick carob
1 C. chopped, locally grown nuts
1 C. chopped, shelled peanuts

½ C. chopped sunflower
    seeds
1½ C. chopped, pitted dates
1 C. grated coconut

Melt the carob and keep warm. In a separate bowl, combine the nuts, peanuts, sunflower seeds, dates, and coconut, and blend well. Shape the mixture into thin cookies. Dip the thin cookies into the warm carob mixture, on both sides, then lay on an oiled pan until the carob becomes firm. Makes about 48 cookies.

Health Cookies

2 C. raw sugar or other
    natural sweetener
½ lb. (2 sticks) butter, softened
3 eggs
2 C. unsweetened coconut

3½ C. whole wheat flour
2 tsp. soda
1½ tsp. cream of tartar
1 cup sunflower seeds, shelled

Cream together the sugar, butter, and eggs. Add coconut and

blend well. In a separate bowl, combine the flour, soda, and cream of tartar, and add to first mixture. Add the sunflower seeds and mix until well combined. Refrigerate mixture for 1 hour, to make it easier to handle. Pinch off pieces of dough, about a teaspoon at a time, and flatten until almost paper thin, using a wet cloth over a flat-bottom jar or wide glass. Transfer cookies to well-oiled baking sheets and bake at 375° for about 7 to 8 minutes. Makes about 75 cookies.

Fig Fandangos

3 eggs, separated
⅔ C. honey
1 tsp. pure vanilla extract
1 C. nut meats, chopped
1 C. figs, chopped

1 tsp. powdered sea kelp
½ tsp. cinnamon
1 C. peanut flour
3½ C. wheat germ flour

Beat the egg whites and set aside. In a large bowl, combine the egg yolks, honey, vanilla, nut meats, figs, sea kelp, cinnamon, peanut flour, and wheat germ. Then fold in the egg whites. Transfer mixture to a well-oiled 9"x 9" cake pan and bake for about 45 minutes at 350°. Test with a toothpick, making sure the mixture is done before removing from oven. Cool and cut into squares. Remove pieces from pan with a pancake turner or slanted spatula. Makes about 2 dozen.

Coconut Macaroons

2 egg whites
½ tsp. cider vinegar
⅛ tsp. salt

½ C. raw sugar or other
    natural sweetener
½ tsp. vanilla
½ C. coconut, shredded

Beat whites until foamy, then add vinegar and salt. Beat until peaks hold and gradually add sugar, one tablespoon at a time,

beating well after each addition. Lightly fold in vanilla and coconut. Drop by tablespoon onto a cookie sheet. Sprinkle top of
cookies with coconut. Bake at 275° for 20 minutes or until lightly
browned. Makes about 16 cookies.

Uncooked Taffy

½ C. homemade (or   1 C. chopped peanuts, shelled
  unhydrogenated) peanut butter   from whole, unroasted pea-
½ C. honey   nuts
                              Instant soy milk powder

In a bowl, combine the peanut butter, honey, and chopped
peanuts until well blended. Add only enough of the soy milk
powder to make stiff dough. Roll dough into a long roll, place on
a cookie sheet, and chill overnight. In the morning, cut taffy into
1-inch pieces. Makes about 24 pieces.

Lollipops

This recipe makes a healthful treat for children.

1 C. raisins   1 C. figs
1 C. dried prunes   Ground coconut meat, nuts,
1 C. locally grown nut meats   or sunflower seeds (for rolling)
1 C. coconut chunks

Combine the raisins, prunes, nut meats, coconut, and figs
and run through food grinder or food processor. Shape mixture
into balls, then flatten them into oblongs. Roll each one in either ground coconut meal, ground nuts, or ground sunflower
seeds, and press a wooden lollipop stick into each lollipop.
Makes about 36 to 40 lollipops.

Date-Carob Bars

4 eggs, separated, whites beaten stiff   ¾ C. wheat germ
⅓ C. honey   ⅓ C. carob powder
¾ C. almonds, ground   ¾ C. dates, pitted and chopped

Blend egg yolks with the honey, almonds, wheat germ, carob powder, and dates until well mixed. Fold in the egg whites. Transfer mixture to an oiled 8" x 8" cake pan and bake for about 45 minutes at 325°, or until done. Cut into bars while warm. Makes about 16 bars.

Note: This recipe may be varied by changing the fruit and nuts and by adding different spices with the various combinations.

Candy

1 C. Grandma's Molasses   1 tbs. butter
1 C. raw sugar or other natural sweetener

In a saucepan, combine the molasses, sugar, and butter, and cook slowly for 10 minutes at 270°, as measured with a candy thermometer. Pull until candy becomes light in color.

Date Patties

1 C. dates   Shredded coconut or
1 C. pecans   chopped nuts (for rolling)

Combine dates and pecans in a food processor and mix thoroughly. Form into patties and roll in coconut or chopped nuts. Makes about 16 patties.

Natural Candy Bars

1 lb. black Mission figs   Chopped nuts (for rolling)
2 C. almonds

Combine figs and almonds in a food processor until well blended. Roll out to ½ inch thickness on wax paper to prevent sticking to board. Cut into bars 3 inches long and 1 inch wide. Cover each bar with chopped nuts and wrap in wax paper. Makes about 2 dozen bars.

Raisin Balls

1 lb. raisins   Freshly grated coconut

Grind raisins in a food processor. Form into balls and roll in freshly grated coconut. Makes about 36 balls.

Fig Candy

12 white figs   ¼ C. chopped nuts
¾ C. shredded fresh coconut   12 pine nuts
¾ C. sesame seeds

Cut off ¾ inch of the stem end of each fig and open figs for stuffing. Process coconut, sesame seeds, and nuts in a food processor until well combined. Stuff each fig with mixture until full. Garnish each fig with a pine nut. Makes 12.

Carrot Pudding

½ C. butter   1¼ C. whole wheat flour, sifted

¾ C. brown sugar

1 egg

2 tbs. water

¾ C. raw carrots, grated

⅓ C. dates, chopped

½ C. seedless raisins

2 tbs. lemon peel, finely chopped

1 tsp. baking powder

½ tsp. salt

⅓ tsp. cinnamon

½ tsp. nutmeg

⅛ tsp. allspice

½ C. nuts, chopped

Cream together butter and sugar until light and fluffy, add egg and water, and beat thoroughly. Add carrots, dates, raisins, nuts, and lemon peel, and blend well. Sift together flour, baking powder, salt, cinnamon, nutmeg, and allspice, and gradually add to creamed mixture. Turn into buttered 5-cup mold. Bake for 1¼ to 1½ hours at 325°. Allow to stand for 5 minutes and remove from mold. Serve warm. Serves 8 to 10.

Note: Pudding may be prepared ahead of time and refrigerated or frozen. To reheat, wrap in foil and place in oven until heated through.

Fruit Crumb Pudding

2 C. whole wheat crumbs

2 C. hot milk

1½ C. mixed raisins, dates, and figs

1 egg, beaten

Mix crumbs in hot milk and let stand for 10 minutes. Steam mixed raisins, dates, and figs for 5 minutes. Add to bread crumbs. Then add egg and mix thoroughly. Transfer to an oiled baking dish and bake at 350° for 30 minutes. Serves 4 to 6.

Date Cream

1 C. dates, pitted

1 C. applesauce

1½ C. whipped cream

Mash dates, mix with applesauce, and add whipped cream. Pile into sherbet glasses and chill. Serves 4 to 6.

Date Coconut Cream

1 C. dates, pitted and ground   2 C. whipped cream
½ C. fresh coconut

Combine dates, coconut, and whipped cream and chill thoroughly. Serves 4 to 6.

Vanilla Rice Custard

3 tbs. natural brown rice, unpolished   ½ C. raisins (optional)
1 C. milk, skim or whole   1 egg, beaten slightly
3 tbs. dark brown sugar   Nutmeg
1 tsp. vanilla

In a bowl, combine the brown rice, milk, sugar, vanilla, raisins, and egg, mixing thoroughly. Transfer to an oiled casserole dish and sprinkle nutmeg over top. Bake in 325° oven for about 1 hour or until a knife comes out clean after testing. Serves 4.

Coconut Custard

3 eggs, beaten   2 C. coconut milk
⅓ C. honey   ¼ tsp. mace
1 tsp. pure vanilla   Fresh grated coconut (for garnish)

In a bowl, combine the eggs, honey, vanilla, coconut milk, and mace. Beat well and pour into a small baking dish. Set this in a pan of hot water and bake in a 325° oven until the custard is set in the center, about 1 hour. Cool, then grate fresh coconut over the top and serve. Serves 4.

Coconut Rice

1 egg yolk
1 tsp. honey
½ C. shredded fresh coconut

½ C. chopped almonds
½ C. coconut milk
1 C. boiling hot brown rice

In a bowl, blend the egg yolk, honey, coconut, almonds, and coconut milk, and stir into a saucepan with the hot rice. Mix well, then remove from heat and allow to cool. Serves 4.

Glorified Rice

1 C. brown rice, cooked
1 C. crushed pineapple, drained
⅓ C. honey

½ tsp. salt
1 C. whipped cream

In a bowl, combine the brown rice, pineapple, honey, and salt until well blended. Fold in the whipped cream. Serves 4.

Dried Apricots in Gelatin

¾ C. dried apricots
Hot water to cover apricots
1 pkg. (small) peach gelatin

1 C. boiling water to
    dissolve gelatin
¼ C. yogurt

Soak apricots in hot water and allow to cool a few hours or overnight. Purée apricots in blender and add peach gelatin made with the boiling water. Put one half of the mixture from the blender into a bowl or mold and let stand until it sets, about 10 minutes. Then either mix in the yogurt or spread it on top of mixture in bowl, and cover with remaining blender mixture. Serves 4.

Lemon Cream Gelatin Dessert or Salad

1 pkg. unflavored gelatin
1 C. natural sugar
Juice of 1 lemon (about 2 tbs.)
1 C. crushed, unsweetened pineapple,
    drained with juice reserved

1½ C. hot water
½ C. Cheddar cheese, grated
½ pt. whipped cream

Combine the gelatin with the sugar and lemon juice. Add the reserved pineapple juice and the hot water and stir until gelatin is dissolved. Chill mixture until gelatin begins to set. Then add the crushed pineapple and grated cheese, and fold in the whipped cream. Return to refrigerator to chill. Serves 4 to 6.

Strawberry Ice

2 C. fresh, hulled strawberries
2 egg yolks

½ C. honey
1 C. fresh pineapple juice

In a blender combine the strawberries, egg yolks, honey, and pineapple juice. When blended, pour the mixture into a freezing tray and stir it several times while it freezes. Serves 4.

Honey Freeze

6 eggs, separated
½ tsp. salt
1½ C. honey

1 envelope unflavored gelatin
Whipped cream (for garnish)
Chopped pistachio nuts (for
    garnish)

Beat egg yolks until thick and lemon colored. Combine with salt, honey, and gelatin in the top of a double boiler. Cook over boiling water, stirring constantly, until mixture is somewhat thickened and smooth. Cool mixture in a pan of ice water until thoroughly chilled. Beat egg whites until soft peaks form. Gently fold egg yolk mixture into egg whites. Pour mixture into freezer trays or individual molds. Freeze for 2 hours. Serve with garnish of whipped cream and nuts. Makes about 1½ quarts.

French Strawberry Pie

1 (3 oz.) pkg. cream cheese
2 baskets strawberries
1 baked pie shell
3½ tbs. cornstarch

1¼ C. unrefined sugar
1 tbs. lemon juice
⅓ C. whipping cream, whipped
 (for garnish)
Food coloring (optional)

Spread softened cream cheese in bottom of pie shell and press ½ of the choicest berries, whole, into the cheese, tips up. Mash remaining berries. Measure to make 1½ cups berries and juice (add water if necessary). Mix cornstarch and sugar, add berries and lemon juice, and cook until thick. Add a few drops food coloring, if desired, and cool. Pour mixture over pie shell containing cream cheese and strawberries. Chill 4 hours. Serve garnished with whipped cream. Serves 8.

6

Beverages

Milk was frequently recommended in the readings, especially certified raw milk. The use of raw milk runs contrary to the opinions in many health magazines and books, but most nutritionists recognize the importance of milk for its protein and calcium content. Soy and nut milk recipes are included here for the benefit of those who may be allergic to cow's milk or simply prefer not to drink it. Soy and nut milks supply most of the nutritional elements of cow's milk, but without the saturated fat and cholesterol.

Since chocolate is now deemed generally detrimental to health, recipes are given using carob, a chocolate substitute, along with other ingredients both pleasing to the taste and healthful from the viewpoint of the readings.

Raw vegetable juices have most of the nutritional value of the vegetables from which they are prepared and can be taken in much larger quantities than would be possible with the whole vegetable. Since roughage is important in the diet, we suggest adding the juice rather than substituting it for the raw fresh vegetables. One individual was advised by the readings to take vegetable juices, either separately or in combination, once or twice a week (1709-10). Another was told to take an ounce of raw carrot juice at least once a day. Vegetable juices are available at supermarkets and health food stores or can be prepared at home with a vegetable juicer.

Fruit juices as beverages likewise add more of the value of fresh fruit to the diet but should not be substituted for fresh fruit. Citrus fruit juices were those most often recommended in the readings, and it was suggested that lime or lemon juice be added to orange or grapefruit juice (2072-3 and 3525-1) and that lemon and lime juice be combined.

Milk Drinks

Carob Milk Drink #1

2 C. certified whole milk   2 tbs. honey
2 tbs. carob powder   ¼ C. water

Heat milk in a saucepan over medium heat, being careful not to boil. Stir in the carob powder, honey, and water, and stir until well combined. Serves 2.

Carob Milk Drink #2

1 small carob candy bar   Honey, to taste (optional)
2 C. certified whole milk

Melt carob candy in top of double boiler, add milk, and heat until warm, being careful not to boil. Sweeten with honey, if desired. Serves 2.

Carrot Milk

This drink has an attractive carrot tint and a coconutlike flavor.

1 C. certified whole milk   2 medium carrots, cut into
                                          pieces

Place milk and carrots in a blender and liquefy. Serves 2.

Apricot Milk

1 C. ripe raw apricots or   3 C. certified whole milk
  ½ C. cooked dried apricots   Honey, to taste

Place apricots, milk, and honey in a blender and liquefy.
Serves 3 to 4.

Maple-Egg Milk

3 tbs. pure maple syrup   ¼ tsp. pure vanilla
1 egg yolk   Dash of salt
2 C. certified whole milk

In a blender, combine the maple syrup, egg yolk, milk, vanilla,
and salt. Blend ingredients 15 to 20 seconds or until thoroughly
blended. Serves 2.

Yogurt (Bulgarian Buttermilk)

Bulgarian buttermilk, recommended in the Cayce readings
and more commonly known in this country as yogurt, has been
one of the principal foods of the Bulgarians for a long period of
time. It is considered by many to be largely responsible for their
good health, vigor, and virility. Baldness and white hair are said
to be almost unknown in Bulgaria.

The health-giving properties of yogurt are primarily due to
the fact that the bacteria in yogurt (Lactobacillus bulgarius,
Streptococcus lactis, Thermobacterium yogurt) thrive in the in-
testines and are capable of synthesizing large amounts of the

entire group of B vitamins, as well as destroying or inhibiting the action of putrefactive bacteria. The bacteria also partially break down the proteins of the milk, making it more easy to digest, and the acid produced in the milk dissolves some of the calcium, making it more available to the body.

Yogurt may be beaten and served as a beverage, having a flavor very similar to buttermilk. If the taste is not enjoyable at first, a taste for it may develop gradually by having it frequently in very small amounts. It may also be served with fruit or berries or as an ingredient in salad dressings.

Basic Yogurt Recipe

Basic recipe: combine 1 quart pasteurized whole or skim milk and ¼ cup commercial yogurt. Warm slowly in oven, in top of double boiler, or in glasses set in a pan of simmering water on the stove, until milk reaches temperature of 100° to 120°. Maintain temperature between 90° and 120° until milk becomes the consistency of junket, or from 3 to 5 hours. If temperature is kept lower than 90°, lactic acid bacteria, rather than the yogurt culture, will grow; and while these will thicken the milk and are not harmful, they cannot live in the intestinal tract to produce B vitamins. If temperature rises above 120°, the bacteria will be killed and the milk will not thicken.

Thick yogurt: Combine 3 cups pasteurized milk, 1½ cups evaporated milk, and ¼ cup commercial yogurt; or combine 1 quart pasteurized milk, 1 cup powdered skim milk, and ¼ cup yogurt. Proceed as above.

If raw milk is used instead of pasteurized milk, heat to simmering and cool to 120° before adding yogurt starter.

As soon as yogurt has thickened to custard consistency, it should be refrigerated; it may be kept for several days. One-fourth cup of this homemade yogurt may be used instead of commercial yogurt to start the next batch. Yogurt culture may be used, instead, as a starter. It can be obtained from many health food stores.

Grape Buttermilk (or Yogurt) Drink

¼ C. grape juice
2 tbs. lemon juice

2 C. Bulgarian buttermilk,
  or yogurt
2 tbs. honey

In a blender combine the grape juice, lemon juice, yogurt, and honey and blend for about 15 seconds. Serves 2.

Buttermilk (or Yogurt) Drink

2 tbs. honey
1 egg
1 tbs. lemon juice

½ tsp. lemon rind, grated
2 C. Bulgarian buttermilk,
  or yogurt

In a blender, combine the honey, egg, lemon juice, lemon rind, and yogurt and blend for about 20 seconds. Serves 2.

Orange Buttermilk (or Yogurt) Drink

This drink is delicious, even for those who do not care for buttermilk or yogurt.

½ C. orange juice
1½ C. Bulgarian buttermilk, or yogurt

2 tbs. honey
½ tsp. grated orange rind

In a blender, combine the orange juice, yogurt, honey, and orange rind and blend for about 20 seconds. Serves 2.

Pineapple Buttermilk (or Yogurt)

1 C. Bulgarian buttermilk,
  or yogurt

½ C. unsweetened
  pineapple juice

½ C. diced fresh papaya

In a blender combine the yogurt, pineapple juice, and papaya and blend until papaya is liquefied. Serves 2.

Evaporated Milk (for Newborns)

10 oz. Carnation evaporated milk   2 tbs. unpasteurized honey
20 oz. water

Combine the milk, water, and honey until well blended. This will make 30 ounces of formula, which will probably be more than the average newborn needs in 24 hours, until he or she weighs 9 or 10 pounds.

Full-Strength Formula, Evaporated Milk

13 oz. Carnation evaporated milk   3 tbs. unpasteurized honey
19 oz. water

Combine the milk, water, and honey until well blended. This will make about six 5¼-ounce bottles, five 6½-ounce bottles, or four 8-ounce bottles.

Raw Milk Formula (for Newborns)

15 oz. certified whole milk,   3 tbs. unpasteurized honey
    preferably goat's milk   15 oz. "Mineral Cocktail" (see
                                    recipe on p. 139)

Combine the milk, honey, and "Mineral Cocktail" until well blended. This will make 30 ounces of formula. When the child is two or three months old, half the quantity of water would be sufficient for the dilution of the milk. After three months, the milk can be taken straight.

"Mineral Cocktail"

2 C. white potato skins   2 C. water

Boil the potato skins in about 2 cups of water for about 15 to 20 minutes. Strain the liquid into a container, mashing the potato skins against strainer to extract all the liquid. The liquid can then be used as a "mineral cocktail." Makes about 1¾ cups.

Soy Milk Made from Soya Powder

1 C. soya powder   1 tsp. liquid lecithin or
4 C. cold water   1 tbs. salad oil
1 tbs. honey   ¼ tsp. salt

Liquefy the soya powder in the cold water. Let stand for 2 hours, then cook in a double boiler for 1 hour. When cool, liquefy in a blender with the honey, lecithin or oil, and salt. Makes about 1 quart.

Note: This milk is very rich and may be liquefied with seed milks for a wholesome palatable milk at the ratio of 1 cup soy milk to 1 cup nut milk (almond, cashew, etc.).

Soy Milk Made from Soy Flour

1 C. soy flour   1 tbs. liquid lecithin or
2 C. water   ¼ C. salad oil
¼ C. honey   ½ tsp. salt

Liquefy the soy flour in a blender with the water and cook in double boiler for 1 hour over medium heat. When cool, liquefy again in the blender with the honey, lecithin or oil, and salt. If using oil, pour it in gradually, while other ingredients are blending. Add enough water to make 2½ quarts of liquid. This milk may be used in any recipe calling for liquid soy milk. Makes 2½ quarts.

Soybean Milk Made from Whole Soybeans

1 C. raw soybeans   Water (to cover and liquefy)

Soak soybeans for 3 days in the refrigerator, pouring water off each day and adding fresh water. On the third day, pour off water and liquefy the beans with 4 to 5 cups fresh water. Extract all milk by running liquefied beans through a juice press, a fine strainer, or a cloth bag. Put the milk in double boiler and cook for 1 hour. Liquefy again. Makes about 3 cups.

Note: Commercially packaged, fortified soy milks (as well as rice milk and almond milk) are now conveniently available in natural food stores and many supermarkets.

Carob Shake

2 C. soy milk (see previous recipe)   5 pitted dates
2 rounded tbs. carob powder   4 rounded tbs. raw almond
2 tbs. honey   or cashew butter
                                                         2 tbs. pure vanilla

In a blender combine the soy milk, carob powder, honey, dates, nut butter, and vanilla and liquefy ingredients together. Chill and liquefy again. Makes about 3 cups.

Almond Milk (Basic Nut Milk Recipe)

This recipe uses almonds because they are a perfect protein food. However, other nuts such as raw peanuts, pine nuts, sunflower seeds, sesame seeds, Brazil nuts, hazel nuts, or pecans may be used to make this recipe, if desired.

½ C. blanched almonds   Salt, to taste
2 C. water   1 tsp. liquid lecithin
Honey, to taste

In a blender, liquefy the almonds and water, and add honey, salt, and lecithin. Makes about 2½ cups.

Carob and Nut Milk Drink

½ C. raw cashews or almonds   2 tbs. honey
2 C. water   2 tbs. carob powder
¼ C. water

Liquefy the nuts with the 2 cups of water. Heat but do not boil. Pour over a mixture of the ¼ cup water, the honey, and carob powder, stirring until blended. Makes about 3 cups.

Fruit and Vegetable Beverages

Pineapple-Watercress Cocktail

2 C. pineapple juice   1 thick slice of peeled lemon
1 bunch watercress, washed   or 2 tbs. lemon juice
3 tbs. honey   1 C. cracked ice

Combine the pineapple juice, watercress, honey, lemon slice or lemon juice, and cracked ice in a blender until watercress is well puréed and of a drinkable consistency. Serves 4.

Vegetable Cocktail

2 C. tomato juice
1 small celery rib with leaves,
    chopped
2 or 3 sprigs parsley
2 slices lemon, with peel

1 slice green pepper
1 slice onion
¼ tsp. salt
½ tsp. honey
1 C. cracked ice

Mix all ingredients in a blender until vegetables are completely liquefied. Serves 4 to 5.

Pineapple and Alfalfa-Sprouts Drink

2 C. unsweetened pineapple
    juice or orange juice
2 tbs. almond butter

Honey, to taste
1 C. alfalfa sprouts

In a blender, combine the juice, almond butter, honey, and sprouts, and blend until liquefied. Serves 4.

Cranberry Cocktail

2 C. raw cranberries, unsprayed
1 C. water
½ C. honey

Dash of salt
Juice of 1 lime

In a blender, combine the cranberries, water, honey, salt, and lime juice, and blend until liquefied. Strain and chill before serving. Serves 4.

Orange-Coconut Drink

1½ C. shredded coconut
3 C. water
1 small can frozen orange juice

Juice of 1 lime
1 C. cracked ice

In a saucepan, simmer the coconut and water for 10 minutes. Cool, strain, and add the orange juice, lime juice, and cracked ice. Transfer mixture to a blender and blend about 15 seconds or until liquefied. Pour over more cracked ice in tall glasses. Serves 5 to 6.

Raspberry Punch

1½ C. raspberry juice
¼ C. lemon juice
1 C. orange juice
¼ C. lime juice

½ C. honey
½ small cucumber, diced
1 qt. water

In a blender, combine the raspberry juice, lemon juice, orange juice, lime juice, honey, and cucumber, blending until cucumber is liquefied. Let mixture stand in the refrigerator several hours. Then strain and add the water. Makes about 2 quarts.

Boysenberry-Coconut Drink

1½ C. boysenberry juice
¾ C. coconut milk
½ C. orange juice

1 tsp. lime juice
2 tbs. honey

In a blender, combine the boysenberry juice, coconut milk, orange juice, lime juice, and honey, and blend until liquefied. Makes about 3 cups.

Prune-Coconut Drink

1½ C. prune juice   1 tsp. lime juice
½ C. orange juice   1 C. fresh coconut milk

Combine the prune juice, orange juice, lime juice, and coconut milk in a blender and liquefy. Makes 3 cups.

Fruit and Vegetable Juice Combinations (1 pint)

Celery juice	10 oz.	Pineapple juice	8 oz.
Spinach juice	4 oz.	Cabbage juice	8 oz.
Parsley juice	2 oz.	Almond butter	4 tsp.
Carrot juice	11 oz.	Orange juice	8 oz.
Coconut juice	2 oz.	Lime juice	1 oz.
Beet juice	3 oz.	Celery juice	7 oz.
		Almond butter	4 tsp.
Carrot juice	10 oz.		
Beet juice	3 oz.	Celery juice	7 oz.
Spinach juice	3 oz.	Lettuce juice	5 oz.
		Spinach juice	4 oz.
Carrot juice	10 oz.		
Spinach juice	3 oz.	Carrot juice	13 oz.
Mustard greens juice	3 oz.	Coconut juice	3 oz.
Carrot juice	7 oz.	Carrot juice	9 oz.
Celery juice	5 oz.	Beet juice	3 oz.
Lettuce juice	4 oz.	Lettuce juice	4 oz.
Cucumber juice	6 oz.	Carrot juice	7 oz.
Radish juice	5 oz.	Celery juice	4 oz.
Green pepper juice	5 oz.	Parsley juice	2 oz.
		Spinach juice	3 oz.
Coconut milk	8 oz.		
Fig juice	8 oz.	Carrot juice	9 oz.
		Celery juice	5 oz.
Dandelion greens juice	8 oz.	Endive juice	2 oz.
Pineapple juice	8 oz.		

Fruit and Vegetable Juice Combinations (1 pint), cont.

Cucumber juice	3 oz.	Strawberry juice	5 oz.
Watercress juice	3 oz.	Rhubarb juice	5 oz.
Celery juice	3 oz.	Pineapple juice	6 oz.
Tomato juice	4 oz.	Grapefruit juice	8 oz.
Parsley juice	3 oz.	Lemon juice	1 oz.
Orange juice	7 oz.	Spinach juice	3 oz.
Lime juice	1 oz.	Pineapple juice	4 oz.
Pomegranate juice	8 oz.		
4 egg yolks			
Honey	4 tsp.		

7

Soups
and
Broths

*I*t is easier to understand, from a nutritional standpoint, why the readings recommended soups and broths in almost every case where dietary advice was given. Soups and broths are easily digested and when properly prepared contain an abundance of minerals and vitamins. The readings particularly recommended broths of the bony pieces of fowl for their calcium content (808-15), and vegetable soups carrying the marrow of beef bones (1523-8). Gelatin, which the body needs to utilize vitamins (849-75), is extracted by boiling bones for stock. Vegetable parings boiled along with the bones add extra important minerals to the stock, and fresh vegetables added to soups maintain most of their vitamins or minerals.

In making soup stock, bones having bits of meat clinging to them should be browned slowly to develop a more enjoyable flavor, then boiled for 3 or 4 hours or cooked in water in a pressure cooker for ½ hour or longer. Since it is desirable to break down the connective tissue as much as possible, thereby extracting the greatest amount of gelatin and calcium, cooking at high temperatures is preferable to simmering. Adding a small amount of vinegar also hastens the breakdown of connective tissue and increases the amount of calcium and gelatin obtained. The calcium combines with and counteracts the acid. Salt should be added to the water, as this aids in drawing out the juices in the scraps of meat and bones. Vegetable parings should be added only during the last 15 minutes of cooking, and vegetables (added after straining the stock to remove bones and parings) should be finely chopped and cooked quickly in the stock only as long as is necessary for tenderness.

The following recipe for beef juice was given in reading 1343-2 and recommended for several people receiving readings. It was referred to "as medicine . . . " (5374-1) and "almost as medicine . . . " (1100-10) Instructions for eating were explicit:

Take at least a tablespoonful during a day, or two tablespoonsful. But not as spoonsful; rather sips of same. This, sipped in this manner, will work towards producing the gastric flow through the intestinal system . . .   1100-10

Pure Beef Juice

Take a pound to a pound and a half preferably of the round steak. No fat, no portions other than that which is of the muscle or tendon for strength; no fatty or skin portions. Dice this into half inch cubes, as it were, or practically so. Put same in a glass jar without water . . . Put the jar then into a boiler or container with the water coming about half or three fourths toward the top of the jar . . . put a cloth in the container to prevent the jar from cracking. Do not seal the jar tight, but cover the top. Let this boil (the water, with the jar in same) for three to four hours. Then strain off the juice, and the refuse may be pressed somewhat. It will be found that the meat or flesh itself will be worthless. Place the juice in a cool place, but do not keep too long; never longer than three days . . . Hence the quantity made up at the time depends upon how much or how often the body will take this.

1343-2

Basic Soup

Delightful, nutritious soups may be made by adding cooked natural brown unpolished rice to chicken broth, beef broth, or bouillon cubes with fine slivered onions. Just before serving add toasted, buttered croutons.

Chicken Soup with Rice or Noodles

1¼ lb. stewing chicken, cut
   into quarters
1 carrot
2 qt. cold water
1 stalk celery
1 medium onion

2 tsp. salt
¼ tsp. pepper
¼ C. uncooked brown rice
   or whole wheat noodles
2 tbs. minced fresh parsley

Place the chicken, carrot, water, celery, onion, salt, and pepper in a 4½ quart pot. Bring to a boil. Reduce heat to low, cover and simmer approximately 2 hours, or until meat is tender. Remove chicken from pot, strain the liquid, and remove all possible fat. Return the stock to pot, bring to boil, add rice or noodles, cover, and cook until tender. Add parsley. Serves 4 to 6.

Note: To obtain the broth and chicken meat for recipes, proceed with the following. Boil bony pieces of chicken in enough water to cover, to which 1 medium onion has been added. When chicken is tender, remove from heat, cool, and remove meat from bones.

Chicken Soup

2 C. chicken broth (see above note)
1 C. chicken meat (see above note)
1 small can tomatoes
1 C. frozen peas or leftover vegetables

4 celery ribs, diced
1 C. raw cashews
Dash of salt

Place the broth, chicken meat, tomatoes, peas, celery, and cashews in a blender, blending well. Add more broth if desired. Place in saucepan, heat, add salt, and serve. Serves 6 to 8.

Turkey Potato Soup

2 C. turkey or chicken broth	1 small can mushrooms
(prepared as in above recipe)	1 medium potato, with skin
1 C. turkey or chicken meat	Salt, to taste
1 small onion, diced	

Place the broth, meat, onion, mushrooms, and potato in a blender, blending well. Place in saucepan, add salt, heat, and serve. Serves 6.

Fish Broth

Fish head, tail, fins, skin, and bones	Celery stalk with leaves,
Water (to cover)	chopped
1 onion, chopped	Salt and pepper, to taste
½ carrot, chopped	

Place fish parts in a pot and cover with cold water. Add the onion, carrot, and celery, and simmer for about 30 minutes. Strain stock, pressing against strainer with a spoon to extract all the liquid. Season to taste with salt and pepper. Serve as soup, or use in aspic or sauces. The stock may be kept for several days in tightly closed container in the refrigerator. Makes about 1 quart.

Roman Egg Soup

4 C. chicken broth	½ tbs. Parmesan cheese, grated
4 eggs, beaten until thick	⅛ tsp. salt

1½ tbs. whole wheat flour   ⅛ tsp. pepper

Bring chicken broth to boiling point and add egg slowly, until well blended. Continue stirring and add flour, cheese, salt, and pepper. Let simmer for about 5 minutes. Serves 4.

Hot Mushroom Soup

A good take-along choice for lunch, this soup holds up well in a thermos bottle.

2 C. meat or vegetable stock	1 small onion
2 C. mushrooms	1 tsp. marjoram
2 medium potatoes,	1 tbs. cooking oil
scrubbed and cubed	Powdered sea kelp, to taste

In blender or food processor combine the stock, mushrooms, potatoes, onion, and marjoram, and purée. Heat the oil in a saucepan over medium heat, add the soup mixture, season with sea kelp, and simmer about 15 minutes. Serves 4 to 5.

Creamed Alfalfa Sprout Soup

4 C. water	1 tsp. onion powder
¾ C. raw cashew nuts	½ tsp. celery powder
2 tbs. arrowroot powder	2 tbs. vegetable broth powder
1 tbs. whole wheat pastry flour	1 C. alfalfa sprouts
2 tsp. salt	

Combine the water, cashew nuts, arrowroot, flour, salt, onion powder, celery powder, and vegetable broth powder in a blender, then transfer to a saucepan and bring to a boil. Reduce heat to medium and cook until thickened, stirring occasionally. Chop the alfalfa sprouts, approximately ¼ cup to each bowl, and add to soup just before serving. Serves 4.

Parsley Vegetable Broth

1 bunch spinach, chopped
2 C. chopped celery
1 small onion, grated
1 small carrot, grated

Water (to cover)
1 tbs. butter
¼ C. vegetable broth powder
¼ C. chopped fresh parsley

In a pot, combine the spinach, celery, onion, and carrot. Cover with water and cook slowly for 30 minutes. Season with the butter and broth powder, sprinkle with chopped parsley, and serve. Serves 6.

Tomato Soybean Broth

1 small onion, minced
2 small green bell peppers, minced
1 C. cooked soybeans, mashed

4 C. tomato juice
1 tbs. butter

Steam onion and green pepper for 10 minutes. Add the mashed soybeans and tomato juice. Heat but do not boil. Dot with butter and serve. Serves 4 to 5.

Tomato-Almond-Asparagus Soup

4 to 6 cooked asparagus spears
2½ C. canned tomatoes
1 C. raw almonds

1 vine-ripened tomato, if desired
Dash of onion salt
Dash of vegetable salt

Place asparagus, canned tomatoes, almonds, and fresh tomato (if using) in a blender, blending well. Transfer to a saucepan, add onion salt and vegetable salt, and heat but do not boil. Serves 4.

Tomato Cashew Soup

2½ C. canned tomatoes
½ bunch parsley
1 tsp. minced onion

½ C. raw cashews
Dash of vegetable salt

Place the tomatoes, parsley, onion, and cashews in a blender and blend well. Transfer mixture to a saucepan, add vegetable salt, and heat, serving immediately. Serves 4.

Swedish Cucumber Soup

4 C. buttermilk
1 C. sour cream
1 C. diced cucumber
½ C. finely chopped
   cooked beet greens

1 tbs. grated carrot
1 tbs. minced onion
1 tbs. dill
1 tsp. salt
¼ tsp. pepper

Beat buttermilk and sour cream until smooth and add cucumber, beet greens, carrot, onion, dill, salt, and pepper. Simmer gently until vegetables are tender but do not boil. In summer, chill this soup without simmering and serve very cold. Serves 6 to 8.

Tomato and Frozen Pea Soup

4 medium vine-ripened tomatoes
2 large stalks celery
½ C. raw almonds
½ tsp. grated onion

1 pkg. frozen peas, thawed
½ C. water
½ tsp. butter
Dash of salt

In a blender, place the tomatoes, celery, almonds, onion, peas, and water, blending well. Transfer to a saucepan, add butter and salt, and heat. Do not boil. Serve immediately. Serves 6.

8

Menus

Special breakfast, luncheon, and dinner suggestions appeared separately in the readings and are listed together in this chapter. Following these are readings giving a whole day's menu.

Before considering the breakfast suggestions from the readings, remember that in recent years nutritionists have become very concerned about the poor breakfast patterns in this country. They point out that breakfast is extremely important and that a meager breakfast can have a bad effect upon the body's capacity for morning energy. Researchers at Marquette University say that temperatures inside the stomach drop when one is hungry but are quickly restored to normal after eating. At 11 a.m., they say, the poor breakfast-eaters first feel hungry. The temperature drops, and this leads to a lowering of metabolism in the stomach. Accordingly, 11 a.m. is the hour of lowered vitality for many people.

General Suggestions

Mornings—either a whole grain cereal, well cooked, with Milk or cream, *or* citrus fruits. However, *do not* take the citrus fruits *and* the cereals at the same meal; rather alternate these from day to day. Rice cakes, corn cakes or the like, with syrup or honey occasionally, are well to be taken.   2693-1

Mornings—citrus fruit juices, preferably with the pulp; oranges at times, lemons at times, grapefruit at other times. Following this we would have whole wheat toast, or cakes, with milk—and honey as the sweetening . . .

At other periods we would have the cooked whole wheat cereal; or Wheaties, Grape Nuts or any of those that carry a great deal of iron and vitamins for the system.

But do not give the cereals and the fruit juices, or citrus fruit, at the same meal . . .   318-6

Mornings—citrus fruit or stewed fruits (as figs, apples, peaches or the like), but do not serve the stewed fruits with the citrus fruit juices; neither serve the citrus fruits with a dry cereal. When cereals are taken there may be added buckwheat cakes, rice cakes or coddled egg, and a cereal drink. It would be well for these to be altered or changed.   623-1

. . . don't be satisfied with just taking a sandwich . . . use only green vegetables or fresh green vegetables, in the lunch period . . . Not just a scrap of bread and a scrap of meat, or a chocolate soda or milk shake! These are poisons for the system at such periods.   243-17

Noons—would be rather a green vegetable diet, *without* too much bread—rather the brown bread at such times. These may be had with the oils or the dressings; or vegetable soups or meat soups, but none of the heavier foods—and most of this green.   943-11

For lunch, that rather light. Sweets of the fruit juices, or of pies, with milk.   781-1

Noons—especially some raw vegetable; as lettuce, celery, carrots or the like, with preferably vegetable soup . . .   2693-1

Noons—the whole green vegetables, as carrots, cabbage (or slaw), lettuce, celery, spinach and the like. These would be preferably taken with the oil dressings. At this meal there may be also at times taken the meat juices, but no meats.   623-1

Evenings—meat in *moderation,* but no *red* meat; no hog meats at *any* time! though there may be taken at times, *with* eggs, very crisp bacon—but not any grease in it!

... drink plenty of water ...
943-11

... not that this would be all, but merely as an outline ...

Evenings—not too heavy, but fish, fowl or lamb—these *never* fried—and well-cooked vegetables.
2693-1

Evenings, of meats. Not too heavy, and a well balanced vegetable diet, of those that grow above and below the ground.
781-1

In general conditions, we must know that there is a *growing* body; that there is necessarily the usage of the body in its activity, and these energies must be supplied—else we make for a drain upon the whole of the nerve and blood supply of the body. Hence meat should be a portion; not the *greater* portion—each day; not necessarily every single meal, but each day.
759-10

Sample Menus

These would be given in an outline—not the only foods, but an outline:

Mornings—whole grain cereals or citrus fruit juices, though not at the same meal. When using orange juice, combine lime with it. When using grapefruit juice, combine lemon with it ... Egg, preferably only the yolk, or rice or buckwheat cakes, or toast, or just any one of these, would be well of mornings.

Noons—a raw salad, including tomatoes, radishes, carrots, celery, lettuce, watercress—any or all of these, with a soup or vegetable broth, or seafoods ...

Evenings—fruits, as cooked apples; potatoes, tomatoes; fish, fowl, lamb, and occasionally beef but not too often.

Keep these as the main part of a well balanced diet. 1523-17

In the matter of diet itself, we would have this as an outline, though—to be sure—this may be altered from time to time to suit the tastes of the body:

At least three mornings each week we would have the rolled or crushed or cracked whole wheat, that is not cooked too long so as to destroy the whole vitamin force in same, but this will add to the body the proper proportions of iron, silicon and the vitamins necessary to build up the blood supply that makes for resistance in the system. We at other times would have citrus fruits, citrus fruit juices, the yolk of eggs (preferably soft boiled or coddled—not the white portions of same), browned bread with butter, Ovaltine or milk; or coffee, provided there is no milk or cream put in same. Occasionally stewed fruits, as baked apples with cream, stewed figs, stewed raisins, stewed prunes or stewed apricots . . . But do not eat citrus fruits at the same meal with cereals or gruels or any of the breakfast foods . . .

Noons—preferably raw fresh vegetables; none cooked at this meal . . . tomatoes, lettuce, celery, spinach, carrots, beet tops, mustard, onions or the like . . . that make for purifying in the *humor* in the lymph blood . . . We would not take any quantities of soups or broths at this period.

Evenings—broths or soups may be taken in a small measure . . . but let it consist principally of vegetables that are well-cooked and a little of the meats such as lamb, fish, fowl—these are preferable. No fried foods . . .   840-1

Mornings (this is not all to be taken, but as an outline)—citrus fruit juices. When orange juice is taken add lime or lemon juice to same; four parts orange juice to one part lime or lemon. When other citrus fruits are taken, as pineapple or grapefruit, they may be taken as they are from the fresh fruit. A little salt added . . . is preferable . . .

Whole wheat bread, toasted, browned, with butter. Coddled egg, only the yolk of same. A small piece of very crisp bacon if so desired. Any or all of these may be taken.

But when cereals are taken, *do not* have citrus fruits at the same meal . . . Such a combination produces just what we are trying to prevent in the system!

When cereals are used, have either cracked wheat or whole wheat, or a combination of barley and wheat—as in Maltex, if these are desired; or Puffed Wheat, or Puffed Rice, or Puffed Corn—any of these. And these may be taken with certain characters of fresh fruits; as berries of any nature, even strawberries if so desired. (No, they won't cause any of the rash if they are taken *properly!*) Or peaches. The sugar used should only be saccharin or honey. A cereal drink may be had if so desired.

Noons—only raw fresh vegetables. *All* of these may be combined, but grate them—do not eat them so that they would make for that condition which often comes with not the proper mastication. Each time you take a mouthful, even if it's water, it should be chewed at least four to twenty times . . . Each should be chewed so that there is . . . the opportunity for the flow of the gastric forces from the salivary glands well mixed with same. Then we will find that these will make for bettered conditions.

Evenings—vegetables that are cooked in their *own* juices . . . each cooked alone, then combined together afterward if so desired by the body . . . These may include any of the leafy vegetables or any of the bulbular vegetables, but cook them in their *own* juices! There may be taken the meats, if so desired . . . or there may be added the proteins that come from the combination of other vegetables . . . in the forms of certain character of pulse or grains.   3823-3

Mornings—citrus fruits, cereals or fruits . . . or citrus fruits, and a little later rice cakes, or buckwheat or graham cakes, with honey *in* the honeycomb, with milk . . . *preferably* the raw milk *if* certified milk!

Noons—rather vegetable juices than meat juices, with raw vegetables as a salad or the like.

Evenings—vegetables, with such as carrots, peas, salsify, red cabbage, yams or white potatoes—these the smaller variety, with the jackets the better; using as the finishing, or dessert, those of blancmange or jello, or jellies, with fruits—as peaches, apricots, fresh pineapple, or the like. These, as we find, with the occasional sufficient meats for strength, would bring a well-balanced diet.

Occasionally we would add those of the blood building, once or twice a week. The pig knuckles, tripe, and calves' liver, or those of *brains* and the like.   275-24

(Q) Outline diet for three meals a day that would be best for body.

(A) Mornings—citrus fruit juices *or* cereals, but not both at the same meal. At other meals there may be taken . . . others at times, dried fruits or figs, combined with dates and raisins—these chopped very well together. And for this especial body, dates, figs (that are dried) cooked with a little corn meal (a very little sprinkled in), then this taken with milk, should be almost a spiritual food for the body; whether it's taken one, two, three or four meals a day. But this is to be left to the body itself.

Noons—such as vegetable juices . . . and a combination of raw vegetables; but not *ever* any acetic acid or vinegar or the like with same—but oils, if olive oil or vegetable oils, may be used with same.

Evenings—vegetables that are of the leafy nature; fish, fowl or lamb preferably as the meats or their combinations. These of course are not to be all, but this is the *general* outline for the three meals for the body.   275-45

Mornings—whole wheat toast, browned. Cereals with fresh fruits. The citrus fruit juices occasionally. But do not mix the citrus fruit juices *and* cereals at the same meal.

Noons—principally (very seldom altering from these) raw vegetables or raw fruits made into a salad; not the fruits and vegetables combined, but these may be altered. Use such vegetables as cabbage (the white, of course, cut very fine), carrots, lettuce, spinach, celery, onions, tomatoes, radish; any or all of these. It is more preferable that they *all* be grated, but when grated do not allow the juices in the grating to be discarded; these should be used upon the salad itself, either from the fruits or the vegetables. Preferably use the *oil* dressings; as olive oil with paprika . . . Even egg may be included in same, preferably the hard egg (that is, the yolk) and it worked into the oil as a portion of the dressing. Use in the fruit salad such as bananas, papaya, guava, grapes; *all* characters of fruits *except* apples. Apples should only be eaten when cooked; preferably roasted and with butter or hard sauce on same, with cinnamon and spice.

Evenings—a well-balanced cooked vegetable diet, including principally those things that will make for iron assimilated in the system.   935-1

Menus for Children

(Q) Would appreciate outline of an ideal daily diet at this age [six years] and for the near future.

(A) Mornings—whole grain cereals or citrus fruits, but these never taken at the same meal; rather alternate these, using one on one day and the other the next, and so on. Any form of rice cakes or the like, the yolk of eggs and the like.

Noons—some fresh raw vegetable salad, including many different types. Soups with brown bread, or broths, or such.

Evenings—a fairly well coordinated vegetable diet, with three above the ground to one below the ground. Seafood, fowl or lamb; not other types of meats. Gelatine may be prepared with any of the vegetables (as in the salads for the noon meal), or with the milk and cream dishes. These would be well for the body.

3224-2

For a seven-year-old:

Noons . . . a great deal of butter and bread, a great deal of those foods that carry a high calorie content in the carbohydrates—or the sweets, provided they are honey based . . . for these will act with digestive forces in system much better than those of corn or cane sweets.

Evenings—a great deal of the whole vegetables, well-balanced with meats; that is, all the leafy vegetables that agree with the body. And let several of the evening meals each week carry calf's liver, hog tripe or beef tripe, mutton and the like. Do not feed or give the body hog meats . . .

Drink as much milk as the body may well take at such meals.

318-6

For a six-month-old baby:

Do not overcrowd the stomach, or be overanxious as to the amount taken, especially through the hot months. Have plenty of fruit juices—that is, orange juice, preferably—then other juices as the body develops; but do not overcrowd these through the hot months. Make the changes more in the early fall, but do not crowd them too much in the present . . .

Also have plenty of strained oatmeal; but not on the same days, when the orange juice is given. Use preferably the steel cut oats, strained, and with plenty of milk . . .

Yes, owing to the general strength and tendency of the body in the bone structure, there *is* the inclination for not sufficient calcium. Thus it would be well for the body to have the Haliver Oil, rather than the Cod Liver Oil. This . . . in the form of pellets . . . The body will be able to take same without choking, provided it is given at or in the meals.   2289-1

9

More About Cooking, Foods, and Health

Cooking

Steam pressure and waterless cooking are the modern methods advised nowadays for preservation of maximum vitamin and mineral content. The use of Patapar paper accomplishes the same end. A paper of this type, as well as other alternatives, may be obtained from health food stores.

... Keep away from heavy foods. Use those which are body building, as beef juice, beef broth, liver, fish, lamb ... never fried foods. Include butter and milk. Also raw vegetables, and these prepared oft with gelatin. Only the yolk of eggs. Leafy vegetables, raw cabbage and cooked red cabbage, spinach, string beans but not dry beans, not white potatoes and a few of yellow potatoes or yams. Artichokes when in season, only prepared in Patapar Paper, the juices of same mixed with the pulp ...   5269-1

(Q) Consider also the steam pressure for cooking foods quickly ... does it destroy any of the precious vitamins of the vegetables and fruits?

(A) Rather preserves rather than destroys.   462-14

(Q) Does steam pressure cooking at 15 lb. temperature destroy food value in foods?

(A) No. Depends upon the preparation of same, the age, and how long gathered. All of these have their factors in the food values. As it is so well advertised that coffee loses its value in fifteen to twenty to twenty-five days after being roasted, so do foods or vegetables lose their food value after being gathered—in the same proportion in hours as coffee would in days.   340-31

Foods

On the subject of tomatoes, which many people say are too acid for their particular systems, the readings shed considerable light.

(Q) What has been the effect on my system of eating so many tomatoes?

(A) Quite a dissertation might be given as to the effect of tomatoes upon the human system.

Of all the vegetables, tomatoes carry most of the vitamins in a well-balanced assimilative manner for the activities in the system. Yet if these are not cared for properly, they may become very destructive to a physical organism; that is, if they ripen after being pulled, or if there is the contamination with other influences.

In *this* particular body, as we find, the reactions from these have been not *always* the *best*. Neither has there been the normal reaction from the eating of same. For it tends to make for an irritation or humor. Nominally, though, these should form at least a portion of a meal three or four days out of every week; and they will be found to be *most* helpful.

The tomato is one vegetable that in most instances . . . is preferable to be eaten after being canned, for it is then much more uniform.

The reaction in this body, then, has been to form an acid of its own; though the tomato is among those foods that may be taken as the *non*-acid forming.   584-5

(Q) Would it be well for me to eat vegetables such as corn, tomatoes, and the like?

(A) Corn and tomatoes are excellent. More of the [vitamins] are obtained in tomatoes than in any other *one* growing vegetable!   900-386

It is interesting to note that food values given in the readings parallel those available from the USDA. In many instances, the Cayce readings gave nutritional information that modern research verified years later.

(Q) Should plenty of lettuce be eaten?
(A) Plenty of lettuce should always be eaten by most *every* body; for this supplies an effluvium in the blood stream that is a destructive force to *most* of those influences that attack the blood stream. It's a purifier.   404-6

Keep plenty of those foods that supply calcium to the body. These we would find especially in raw carrots, cooked turnips and turnip greens, all characters of salads—especially as of water cress, mustard and the like; these especially taken raw, though turnips cooked—but cooked in their own juices and *not* with fat meats.   1968-6

... often use the raw vegetables which are prepared with gelatin. Use these at least three times each week. Those which grow more above the ground than those which grow below the ground. Do include, when these are prepared, carrots with that portion especially close to the top. It may appear the harder and the less desirable but it carries the vital energies, stimulating the optic reactions between kidneys and the optics.   3051-6

Keep away from sweets, especially chocolate at this period, also foods prepared with coconut. Other characters of nuts are well, though especially almonds are good and if an almond is taken each day, and kept up, you'll never have accumulations of tumors ... An almond a day is much more in accord with keeping the doctor away, especially certain types of doctors, than apples. For the apple was the fall ... the almond blossomed when everything else died.   3180-3

In connection with almonds, which have food values mostly ignored by those in the field of nutrition, it is interesting to note how information from the readings tallies with the latest research and investigation. In Recommended Dietary Allowances by the National Research Council, it is stated that "In the case of other adults the phosphorus allowances should be approximately 1.5 times those for calcium." Almonds are at the top of the list of foods having such a proportion of phosphorus and calcium. Almonds contain 475 mg. of phosphorus, 254 mg. of calcium, and 4.4 mg. of iron. Almonds rank highest in iron of all foods having the proportion of 1.5 times the amount of phosphorus to calcium.

(Q) Please give the foods that would supply [iron, calcium, and phosphorus].

(A) . . . cereals that carry the heart of the grain; vegetables of the leafy kind; fruit and nuts . . . The almond carries more phosphorus *and* iron in a combination easily assimilated than any other nut.   1131-2

In the matter of supplying the calcium and other elements, as phosphorus and salts . . .

At least once or twice a week the sea foods may be taken, especially clams, oysters, shrimp or lobster . . . The oyster or clam should be taken raw . . . the others prepared through roasting or boiling with the butter . . .   275-24

The phosphorous forming foods are principally carrots, lettuce (rather the leaf lettuce, which has more soporific activity than the head lettuce), shell fish, salsify, the *peelings* of Irish potatoes (if they are not too large) . . .   560-2

Vitamins—should we take them separately or in foods? The Cayce readings varied in their advice, apparently according to the individual's body capacity. In the majority of readings, however, the recommendation was to obtain vitamins from foods.

So, keep an excess of foods that carry especially Vitamin B, iron and such. Not the concentrated form, you see, but obtain these from the foods. These would include all fruits, all vegetables that are yellow . . . Thus—lemon and orange juice combined, all citrus fruit juices; pineapple as well as grapefruit. Some of these should be a part of the diet each day.

Squash—especially the yellow; carrots, cooked and raw; yellow peaches; yellow apples (preferably the apples cooked, however).

All of these carry an excess or the greater quantity of necessary elements for suppling energies for the body, and that are much more easily assimilated by the body.

Yellow corn, yellow corn meal, buckwheat—all of these are especially good.

Red cabbage. Such vegetables, such fruits, are especially needed by the body.   1968-7

Knowing the tendencies [toward weakness in your body], supply in the vital energies that ye call the vitamins, or elements. For, remember, while we give many combinations, there are only four elements in your body—water, salt, soda and iodine. These are the basic elements, they make all the rest! Each vitamin as a component part of an element is simply a combination of these other influences, given a name mostly for confusion to individuals, by those who would tell you what to do for a price!   2533-6

All such properties [as vitamins] that add to the system are more efficacious if they are given for periods, left off for periods and begun again. For if the system comes to rely upon such influences wholly, it ceases to produce the vitamins even though the food values may be kept normally balanced.

And it's much better that these be produced in the body from the normal development than supplied mechanically; for nature is much better *yet* than science!

This as we find then, given twice a day for two or three weeks, left off a week and then begun again, especially through the winter months, would be much more effective with the body.

                                                      759-13

(Q) What relation do the vitamins bear to the glands? Give specific vitamins affecting specific glands.

(A) You want a book written on these!

They are food for same. Vitamins are that from which the glands take those necessary influences to supply the energies to enable the varied organs of the body to reproduce themselves. Would it ever be considered that your toenails would be reproduced by the same as would supply the breast, the head or the face? or that the cuticle would be supplied from the same as would supply the organ of the heart itself? These are taken from *glands* that control the assimilated foods, and hence the necessary elements or vitamins in same to supply the various forces for enabling each organ, each functioning of the body to carry on in its creative or generative forces, see?

These will begin with A—that supplies portions to the nerves, to bone, to the brain force itself; not all of this, but this is a part [of the function of A.

B and B-1 supply the ability of the energies, or the moving forces of the nerve and of the white blood supply . . . the brain for itself and the ability of the sympathetic or involuntary reflexes through the body. Now this includes all, whether you are wiggling your toes or your ears or batting your eye, or what! In these we have that supplying to the chyle that ability for it to control the influence of fats . . . (and this body has never had enough of it!), to carry on the reproducing of the oils that prevent the tenseness in the joints, or that prevent the joints from becoming atrophied or dry, or to creak. At times the body has had some creaks!

In C we find that which supplies the necessary influences to the flexes of every nature throughout the body, whether of a muscular or tendon nature, or a heart reaction, or a kidney contraction, or the liver contraction, or the opening or shutting of your mouth, the batting of the eye, or the supplying of the saliva and the muscular forces in face. These are all supplied by C—not that it is the only supply, but a part of same. It is that from which the structural portions of the body are stored, and drawn upon when it becomes necessary. And when it becomes detrimental . . . which has been for this body, it is necessary to supply same in such proportions as to aid; else the conditions become such that there are the bad eliminations from the incoordination of the excretory functioning of the alimentary canal, as well as the heart, liver and lungs, through the expelling of those forces that are a part of the structural portion of the body.

G supplies the general energies, or the sympathetic forces of the body itself.

These are the principles.   2072-9

(Q) What foods carry most of the Vitamin B?

(A) All those that are of the yellow variety, especially, and whole grain cereals or bread.   457-8

In the matter of the diet throughout the periods, we would constantly add more and more of Vitamin B-1, in every form in which it may be taken; in the bread, the cereals, the types of vegetables ... the fruits, etc. Be sure that there is sufficient each day for the adding of the vital energies. These vitamins are not stored in the body as are A, D and G, but it is necessary to add these daily. All of those fruits and vegetables, then, that are yellow in color should be taken; oranges, lemons, grapefruit, yellow squash, yellow corn, yellow peaches ... beets—but all of the vegetables cooked in their *own* juices, and the body eating the juices with same.   2529-1

What are vitamins? One scientist of note remarked that a vitamin is a unit of ignorance—nobody knows what it is, only what it does. Read what these Cayce readings have to say on the subject:

Have ye not read that in Him ye live and move and have thy being? What are those elements in food or in drink that give growth or strength to the body? Vitamins? What are vitamins? The creative forces working with the body-energies for the renewing of the body!   3511-1

Know that the body must function as a unit. For, one may get one's feet wet and yet have cold in the head! One may get the head wet and still have cold in the head! The same is true in any such relationships. For, the circulation carries . . . in the corpuscles, the elements or vitamins needed for assimilation in every organ. For, each organ has within itself that ability to take from that assimilated that necessary to build itself . . .

Hence it may be said that the adding of vitamins to the system is a precautionary measure—at all seasons when the body is the most adaptable or susceptible to the contraction of cold—either by contact or by exposure or from unsettled conditions.   902-1

Remember high school chemistry class, when you added a catalyst to chemicals and watched their reaction speed up? Amino acids seem to be such catalysts. The various kinds of amino acids, when isolated and tested, seem to enable the action of vitamins, making them more useful to the body.

Current scientific interest in amino acids takes on new significance in light of the following Cayce reading on diet and gelatin, which was often mentioned in the readings. In the 1940s, someone asked the sleeping Cayce about gelatin:

(Q) Please explain the vitamin content of gelatin. There is no reference to vitamin content on the package.

(A) It isn't the vitamin content but it is ability to work with the activities of the glands, causing the glands to take from that absorbed or digested the vitamins that would not be active if there is not sufficient gelatin in the body. See, there may be mixed with any chemical that which makes the rest of the system susceptible or able to call from the system that needed. It becomes then, as it were, "sensitive" to conditions. Without it there is not that sensitivity.   849-75

According to the Knox Gelatin Company, "No one food article supplies all of the types of amino acids that make up the complete protein . . . Real gelatin and several of the cereal and vegetable proteins are in this class. Unflavored gelatin which contains 9 of the 10 essential amino acids takes its place as a useful supplementary protein . . . The protein of real gelatin contains amino acids that have special value in the production of hemoglobin."

According to Evelyn Roehl in *Whole Food Facts* (Inner Traditions, 1996), "In order for our bodies to make use of the protein we consume, these essential amino acids must be present in the digestive system simultaneously and in specific proportions. When they are, our bodies create complete proteins."

Not too heavy a diet; that is, not too much meats, more vegetables. Fruits and nuts may be included . . . Raw vegetables prepared oft with gelatin. Gelatin, ices, ice cream; all of these may be taken.   3395-4

Do not leave off the gelatin. Do keep the vitamins that will add strength to the body.   3389-1

Do have raw vegetables oft. These not as to cause too great a relaxation, but those energies as with the nerve-building forces from celery, lettuce, tomatoes, carrots—but grate or chop fine. Oft prepare these with gelatin.   5390-1

In the diet keep plenty of raw vegetables, such as watercress, celery, lettuce, tomatoes, carrots. Change these in their manner of preparation, but do have some of these each day. They may be prepared rather often with gelatin, as with lime or lemon gelatin—or Jello. These will not only taste good but be good for you.   3429-1

Have a great deal of such as liver, tripe, pigs' knuckle, pigs' feet and the like; a great deal of okra and its products, a great deal of any form of desserts carrying quantities of gelatin. Any of the gelatin products, though they may carry sugars at times, these are to be had oft in the diet.   2520-2

In building up the body with foods, preferably have a great deal of raw vegetables for this body, as lettuce, celery, carrots, watercress. All should be taken raw, with dressing, and oft with gelatin. These should be grated, or cut very fine, or even ground, but do preserve all of the juices with them when these are prepared in this manner in the gelatin.   5394-1

Health

The Cayce readings recommended that everyone consume food that is grown locally, particularly those individuals who wish to acclimate, or adjust, to a new environment. While this concept has not been scientifically defined nor have difficulties or diseases been traced to the lack of it, those who travel to different parts of the country—or even a few miles beyond home territory—often complain of the upset caused by a change in drinking water. Such an upset may just as easily be caused by a change of food grown in another locality, reacting differently in the body. It is important to note that frozen foods, vegetables, meats, and seafoods native to specific regions are widely used in many other sections of the country.

The Cayce readings gave definite advice on the subject of acclimatization:

(Q) Is the climate of . . . Texas satisfactory and should I remain here?

(A) The climatic conditions here are not the basis of the trouble. The body can adjust itself. As we have indicated bodies can usually adjust themselves to climatic conditions if they adhere to the diet and activities, or all characters of foods that are produced in the area where they reside. This will more quickly adjust a body to any particular area or climate than any other thing.

(Q) Is a diet composed mainly of fruits, vegetables, eggs, and milk the best diet for me?

(A) As indicated, use more of the products of the soil that are grown in the immediate vicinity. These are better for the body than any specific set of fruits, vegetables, grasses or what not. We would add more of the original source of proteins.   4047-1

[Have] vegetables that are fresh, and as are *especially* grown in the vicinity where the body resides. Shipped vegetables are never very good.   2-14

Have raw vegetables also, but not a great deal of melons of any kind, though cantaloupes may be taken if grown in the neighborhood where the body resides; if shipped don't eat it. The fruits that may be taken: plums, pears and apples. Do not take raw apples, but roast apples a plenty.   5097-1

Do not have large quantities of any fruits, vegetables, meats, that are not grown in or come to the area where the body is at the time it partakes of such foods. This will be found to be a good rule to be followed by all. This prepares the system to acclimate itself to any given territory.   3542-1

Water

Do you drink enough water? Most people do not drink as much as they think—or say—they do. Some health information sources recommend drinking six to eight glasses of water a day, exclusive of juices, tea, coffee, etc.; others lower this to four to six glasses. Is drinking water important? The Cayce readings say it is.

... there should be more water taken in the system in more consistent manner, that the system, especially in the hepatics and kidneys, may function more nominally, thus producing the correct manner for eliminations of drosses in system, for ... there are many channels of elimination from system. For this reason each channel should be kept in that equilibrium, or in that balance wherein the condition is not brought to an accentuated condition in any *one* of the eliminating functioning conditions; not overtaxing lungs, not overtaxing the kidneys, not overtaxing the liver, not overtaxing the respiratory system, but all kept in that equal manner ...

The lack of this water in system creates, then, the excess of those eliminations, that should nominally be cleansed through alimentary canal and through the kidneys, back to the capillary circulation ...   257-11

Well to drink *always plenty* of water, before meals and after meals—for, as has oft been given, when any food value *enters* the stomach *immediately* the stomach becomes a storehouse, or a medicine chest that may create all the elements necessary for proper digestion within the system. If this *first* is acted upon by aqua pura, the reactions are more near normal. Well, then, each morning upon first arising, to take a half to three-quarters of a glass of *warm* water; not so hot that it is objectionable, not so tepid that it makes for sickening but this will clarify the system of poisons.   311-4

(Q) How much water should I drink daily?
(A) From six to eight tumblers full.   574-1

Sleep

Few of us get enough sleep or as much as we think we need in order to feel at our best. If we deliberately deprive ourselves of enough sleep, this can eventually take its toll on the body. The readings say, "Take time to sleep!"

Take *time* to sleep! It *is* the exercising of a faculty, a condition that is meant to be a part of the experience of each soul. It is as but the shadow of life, or lives, or experiences, as each day of an experience is a part of the whole that is being builded by an entity . . . And each night is as but a period of putting away, storing up into the superconscious or the unconsciousness of the soul itself.

                                                               2067-3

Seven and a half to eight hours should be [taken] for *most* bodies.   816-1

Sedatives or hypnotics . . . are rather destructive forces to brain and nerve reflexes.   3431-1

(Q) Why can't I sleep at night?
(A) This is from nervousness and overanxiety. Of course, keep away from any drugs if possible—though a sedative at times may be necessary.
Drink a glass of warm milk with a teaspoonful of honey stirred in same.   2514-7

(Q) What may be done to enable me to sleep through the night?
(A) Purifying of the system in the manners indicated will relieve the tensions upon the nervous system . . .
For . . . if the body takes the time for thought—physical rest is the natural means of the mental and spiritual finding the means of coordinating with the activities of the mental-physical in the

body . . . Hence rest is necessary, but that which would be *induced*—unless it becomes necessary because of pain or the like—is not a *natural* rest, nor does it produce a regeneration for the activities of the physical body.   1171-1

(Q) Why am I so dependent upon sleep, and what do I do during my physical sleep?

(A) Sleep is a *sense*, as we have given heretofore; and is that needed for the physical body to recuperate, or to draw from the mental and spiritual powers or forces that are held as the ideals of the body.

Don't think that the body is a haphazard machine, or that the things which happen to individuals are chance . . .

Then, what happens to a body in sleep? Dependent upon what it has thought, what it has set as its ideal! For, when one considers, one may find these as facts! There are individuals who in their sleep gain strength, power, might—because of their thoughts, their manner of living. There are others who find that when any harm, any illness, any dejection comes to them, it is following sleep! It is again following a law!

What happens to this body? Dependent upon the manner it has applied itself *during* those periods of its waking state.

2067-3

Smoking, Coffee, and Tea

Is smoking compatible with everyday living in which a strong effort is made to apply ideals? What about alcoholic drinks, coffee, and tea? Are they harmful? Information given in the readings is extremely helpful.

(Q) Have personal vices as tobacco and whiskey any influence on one's health or longevity?

(A) . . . you are suffering from the use of some of these in the present; but it is over-indulgence. In moderation these are not too bad, but man so seldom will be moderate. Or, as most say, those who even indulge will make themselves pigs, but we naturally are pigs when there is over-indulgence. This, of course, makes for conditions which are to be met. For what one sows that must one reap. This is unchangeable law.   5233-1

(Q) Does smoking hurt the body?
(A) Moderation, not so harmful as would be the nerve and
mental reaction from total abstinence from same.
Then, a moderation.   1568-2

(Q) Would smoking be detrimental to me or beneficial?
(A) This depends very much upon self. In moderation, smoking is not harmful; but to a body that holds such as being out of
line with its best mental or spiritual unfoldment, do not smoke.
                                                      2981-2

(Q) Is the moderate use of liquor, tobacco and meat a bar to
spiritual growth?
(A) For this entity, yes. For some, no.   2981-1

. . . wine taken in excess—of course—is harmful; wine taken
with bread alone is body, blood and nerve and brain building.
                                                      821-1

No beer, no strong drink; though red wine as a *food* may be
taken occasionally—for this is blood building and blood-resist-
ing forces are carried in same—as iron and those plasms that
make for the proper activity upon the system. But never more
than two or two and a half ounces of same, but this only with
black or brown bread, and not with sweets.   1308-1

(Q) Is too much coffee and smoking dangerous for his nerves
or stomach?
(A) Not necessarily. Depends upon how it is prepared. With
milk it is very dangerous.
Smoking in moderation is not harmful . . .   3477-1

(Q) Will coffee hurt the body?
(A) Coffee without cream or milk is not so harmful. Preferably
the G. Washington Coffee, because of its *manner* of brewing.
                                                      1568-2

(Q) Is coffee good? If so, how often?

(A) Coffee taken properly is a food value.

To many conditions, as with this body, the caffeine in same is hard upon the digestion; especially where there is the tendency for a plethora condition in the lower end of the stomach.

Hence the use of coffee or the chicory . . . from the *combinations* of coffee with breads or meats or sweets helpful.

But for this body, it is *preferable* that the tannin be mostly removed. Then it can be taken two or three times a day, but *without* milk or cream. 404-6

. . . coffee is . . . as stimulants to the nerve system. The dross from same is caffeine, as is not digestible in the system, and must necessarily then be eliminated. When such are allowed to remain in the colon, there is thrown off from same poisons. Eliminated as it is in this system, coffee is a food value, and is preferable to many stimulants that might be taken . . . 294-86

(Q) Does it hurt me to use sugar in my coffee?

(A) Sugar is not near so harmful as cream. May use sugar in moderation. 243-22

(Q) Are tea and coffee harmful?

(A) For this body tea is preferable to coffee, but in excess is hard upon the digestion. To be sure, it should never be taken with milk. 1622-1

(Q) Is tea and coffee harmful to the body?

(A) Tea is more harmful than coffee. Any nerve reaction is more susceptible to the character of tea that is usually found in this country, though in some manners in which it is produced it would be well. Coffee, taken properly, is a food; that is, *without* cream or milk. 303-2

Recreation

Work, rest, recreation, exercise, elimination, food, and drink—all these are the physical factors of life having mental and spiritual effects that must be balanced with the time we take for the purely spiritual. The difficulties of reaching this proper balance—different for each individual—are reflected in the following questions put to Edgar Cayce, and the wonderfully constructive answers.

We find that these [conditions] arose as a result of what might be called occupational disturbances; not enough in the sun, nor enough of hard work. Plenty of brain work, but the body is supposed to coordinate the spiritual, mental and physical. He who does not give recreation a place in his life, and the proper tone to each phase—well, he just fools self . . . There must be certain amounts of rest. These are physical, mental and spiritual necessities. Didn't God make man to sleep at least a third of his life? Then consider! This is what the Master meant when He said, "Consider the lilies of the field, how they grow." Do they grow all the while, bloom all the while, or look mighty messy and dirty at times? It is well for people, individuals, as this entity, to get their hands dirty in the dirt at times, and not be the white-collared man all the while! . . . From whence was man made? Don't be afraid to get a little dirt on you once in a while . . .

And take time to play a while with others. There are children growing. Have you added anything constructive to any child's life? You'll not be in heaven if you're not leaning on the arm of someone you have helped.   3352-1

(Q) Do you advise the use of colonics or Epsom Salts baths for the body?
(A) When these are necessary, yes. For *every* one—everybody—should take an internal bath occasionally, as well as an external one. They would all be better off if they would!   440-2

Clear the body as you do the mind of those things that have hindered. The things that hinder physically are the poor eliminations. Set up better eliminations in the body. This is why osteopathy and hydrotherapy come nearer to being the basis of all needed treatments for physical disabilities.   2524-5

For the hydrotherapy and massage are preventive as well as curative measures. For the cleansing of the system allows the body-forces themselves to function normally, and thus eliminate poisons, congestions and conditions that would become acute through the body.   257-254

(Q) What physical and mental exercises will be beneficial?

(A) Of course, a meditation is well always; for the mental attitude has much to do with the general physical forces.

As for the physical exercises, walking is the best of any exercise—and swimming, now for the next three to four months.
2823-2

The exercise that we would follow for this body would be the stretching much in the manner as the exercise of the cat or the panther ... stretching the muscular forces, not as strains but as to cause the tendons and muscles to be put into position for the formation of strength-building to the body.   4003-1

(Q) Is there any special exercise I should take, other than the head and neck exercise?

(A) Walking is the best exercise, but don't take this spasmodically. Have a regular time and do it, rain or shine!   1968-9

(Q) Has lack of setting-up exercises in last months been detrimental to the body?

(A) Whenever something is begun and then left off, it becomes detrimental—that should have been kept up!   457-12

... fasting ... is as the Master gave: Laying aside thine own concept of *how* or *what* should be done at this period, and let the Spirit guide. Get the truth of fasting! The body, the man's bodily functioning, to be sure, *overdone* brings *shame* to self, over indulgence in anything—but the true fasting is casting out of self that as "I would have done," [replacing with] "but as *Thou*, O Lord, seest fit—use me as the channel, as the strength comes by the concerted and cooperative seeking of many to give Thy strength to a body!"   295-6

Take time to be holy, but take time to play also. Take time to rest, time to recuperate; for thy Master, even in the pattern in the

earth, took time to rest, took time to be apart from others . . .
took time to attend a wedding, to give time to attend a funeral;
took time to attend those awakenings from death and took time
to minister to all.   5246-1

Index

187